1000
BEST TIPS FOR
ADHD

Expert Answers and Bright Advice to Help You and Your Child

SUSAN ASHLEY, PhD

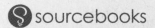
sourcebooks

Published by Sourcebooks, Inc.
P.O. Box 4410, Naperville, Illinois 60567-4410
(630) 961-3900
Fax: (630) 961-2168
www.sourcebooks.com

CIP data is on file with the publisher.

Printed and bound in the United States of America.
VP 10 9 8 7 6 5

Dedication

For Lanterne Rouge. You may come in last, but you always cross the finish line.

Contents

Acknowledgments

Creating *1,000 Best Tips for ADHD* did not happen quickly. It is an accumulation of experience gained in twenty-five years of working with hundreds of families living with ADHD. While my education and training provided the foundation for my knowledge about ADHD, it is my work in the psychological trenches with children and their families that allowed me to create, test, and verify the tips in this book. Getting to know each child and family individually, learning how they operate in their lives, discovering their likes and dislikes, their capabilities and limitations, they allowed me to design techniques and solutions customized for them. Through trial and error, together we would find which tips were effective for their situation. I wish to thank the many families with whom I have had the joy of sharing success in managing the symptoms of ADHD.

I owe many thanks to my editor, Kelly Bale, for her vision in the development of this book. Sabrina Baskey-East, Heather Hall, and Regan Fisher were invaluable with their keen eye for detail.

As always, gratitude to my parents, who provided me with a solid foundation in childhood, unknowingly using many parenting techniques I would later bring to my practice in psychology.

Forever, my deepest appreciation to Stan for every little thing.

Introduction

How do I get my child to do his homework? How can I make her brush her teeth without arguing with me every night? What do I do when he lies about the same thing over and over? Why doesn't punishment seem to make any difference? *1000 Best Tips for ADHD* is your go-to guide for the challenges your child presents. In this book, you will find the answers to these problems and most other situations you face raising a child with ADHD.

Raising a child with ADHD is tough, really tough. When faced with a problem or impossibly frustrating situation, you want answers, and you want them fast. Here they are! Quick, easy to read, and easy to put into action, *1000 Best Tips for ADHD* lets you look up specific answers to the exact problems you are facing and find ways to implement immediate solutions. Because no two children with ADHD are alike, you will not find the usual one-solution-fits-all approach in this book. Instead, you will find a multitude of options so that you can find the one that works best for your child.

And because, as a parent of a child with ADHD, you know

that what worked today may not work tomorrow, *1000 Best Tips for ADHD* gives you many different ways to solve each problem so that when one solution stops working, you will turn back to this book and find dozens of other options.

As a child psychologist specializing in ADHD for more than twenty years, I know exactly what parents are facing every day. Your child has numerous behaviors that are challenging for both you and for her. No two days are alike. Life with an ADHD child is consistently inconsistent, predictably unpredictable. Simply getting through the ordinary tasks of the day can be a relentless challenge that never seems to get easier. *1000 Best Tips for ADHD* will give you the tools you need to make the days go smoother so you and your child stop the battles over behavior and can have the happier, emotionally rewarding relationship you both deserve.

How to Use This Book

1000 Best Tips for ADHD is a how-to manual that is easy to use. It does not require you to read it cover to cover. You can look in the table of contents to find the problem you are trying to manage, turn to the chapter, and find many different solutions. No one tip is better than another. Read each solution, select one you think might work, and give it a try.

Keep a daily log of how it went so you can keep track of the ones that worked and those that did not. If the solution works, keep doing it until it is no longer effective. ADHD children change rapidly, and a solution that works for several weeks or months may lose its effectiveness and require you to come up with a new one. This is not a problem! I know that at some point, whatever solution you initially pick might wear off, so I have given you many other possible solutions. Go back to the chapter, find another solution, and give it a try. It's that simple.

1000 Best Tips for ADHD gives you the many hundreds of solutions I have used in my twenty-plus years in private practice working with families living with ADHD. Each of the thousand tips has been tested and verified to work by the hundreds of families I have helped in my practice. These are the strategies I would suggest to you if you brought your child to my office. We would identify the problem your child is having, and I would suggest the one solution I thought would be most successful. I would ask you and your family to try it for one week while keeping a daily journal of who, where, what, when, why, and how you used the tip.

I would go over the journal with you, and together we would determine if the solution was a success. We would need to make sure, however, that you used it in the proper way and that you did so consistently, every day, and did not change it in any way. Too often parents will tell me "It didn't work!" Despite their promises that they did it perfectly, when we really dissect what they did, the failure is not due to the tip itself, but rather that the parents did not use the strategy properly.

Before you conclude that the solution you tried was ineffective, imagine you are sitting with me in my office and we are analyzing how skillful you were in using it. We do this because I know without a doubt that every solution I have given you in this book works. I also know it is all too easy for parents to blame the solution and hope for a different one that will be easier and take less time and effort to implement. I know you will think this applies to other parents and not to you, but trust me, it applies to all parents. No one wants to admit that a child's behavior problems have anything to do with the parenting. I do not want parents to think about blame, but for children to behave better, parents need to understand that how they parent does affect their child's behavior. Parents do not cause ADHD, but they can make it better or worse.

If you know without a doubt that you tried the tip with near perfection, and it did not result in a positive change, then go ahead and feel confident in trying another one.

The tips are written in no particular order, so use your intuition about your child to feel what might work best. If you work full-time, do not get home until 7:00 p.m., and have three kids to feed, help with homework, bathe, and get ready for bed, then do not pick a solution that involves you having an hour of playtime each night with your child as his reward for a good day at school. Be realistic about what you can and cannot do, and pick solutions that fit your life. This is the beauty of *1000 Best Tips for ADHD*: one size definitely does not fit all. You can pick and choose what fits for you and your child.

How Do I Tell If a Tip Is Working?

The most important way to tell if a tip is working is to define what to expect. Too many parents expect a cure, and if not a cure, then at least for the behavior to stop. If the child is not cured or does not stop the problematic behavior, parents conclude that the solution did not work and they go on an endless search for the magic pill or magic technique that will "work."

Many parents' expectations are too high for the reality of ADHD. Perhaps it is because they have been sold the dream by the pharmaceutical advertisements of the smiling mommy next to her child brimming with pride, holding his A+ homework. Parents are told that medication is "effective" for 80 percent of the children who take it, yet they are not told what "effective" means. Parents assume "effective" means "it works" just like other medicines: take a pill, feel better, problem over.

Not so with ADHD. Nothing cures ADHD. Children who have ADHD will have symptoms, at a minimum, through their childhood years, and most likely through adolescence. It is not going away, and no pill will cure it. Nor will any psychological technique, tool, or tip you use.

Expectations for what is effective and what works for ADHD have to be brought in line with the reality of the disorder. The harsh reality is that it is not curable. Nothing you do is going to stop it. But everything you do can manage it. Your goal is to use the tips in this book to manage the symptoms. If a tip helps manage ADHD symptoms, it is effective. If you stop using the tip, chances are the symptom will worsen.

The goal with ADHD is to decrease how often, how intense, how long, and how disruptive the symptoms are. If you use a tip and the problem happens less often, is less severe, and causes fewer negative consequences, then that tip is effective. Over the years—yes, years—the problem will likely go away as your child builds skills of her own, but we are talking years, not weeks or months.

Parents who understand that their children's ADHD is here to stay and who focus on learning how to live with the disorder, rather than fighting it, have a far easier time of it. They focus on making life as smooth as possible, given the presence of ADHD in their lives. They do not live in frustration and disappointment. They embrace their children and use various tips to live *with* ADHD.

The more you know about ADHD, the easier it is to accept the presence of this uninvited disorder into your life. A solid understanding of ADHD, what it is, what it isn't, what other disorders coexist with it, as well as how to get an evaluation, what medication can and cannot do, and much more can be found in *The ADD & ADHD Answer Book: Professional Questions to 275 of the Top Questions Parents Ask*. With greater knowledge about the disorder, you will be in a better position to understand the why and the how of the tips presented in this book.

An understanding of a token economy/point system will enhance your ability to use many of the tips in this book. Throughout the book, you will see that I recommend the use of points to reward your child for cooperation. A token economy is a system where your child earns a fixed number of points for each task completed. You may also hear it referred to as a behavior chart or point system. While a behavior chart may include a few behaviors, a token economy is a more comprehensive plan where your child earns points or tokens, such as poker chips, for almost every behavior required of him. Getting out of bed, getting dressed, brushing teeth, eating breakfast, and so on, including the remainder of tasks he engages in from the time he wakes up to the time he goes to bed, are rewarded with points or tokens. The points or tokens are exchanged for privileges, such as watching television or having a sleepover; favorite foods such as pizza or ice cream sundaes; and prizes such as stickers, toys, clothes, games, and countless other desirable items. ADHD children with only a few behavior problems will do well with a simple behavior chart targeting the three to four behaviors they struggle with. Those with a more severe form of ADHD will do better with a token economy that targets their activities, tasks, and behaviors throughout the day and night.

Getting Started

Tips for DIAGNOSIS

Your child has most likely already been diagnosed; otherwise, you probably would never have picked up this book. However, there is more to diagnosis than just ADHD. These twenty-one tips will help you determine if your child needs additional evaluation.

1. Be sure that your child has been evaluated by a child psychologist, not just a pediatrician or psychiatrist. A child psychologist can determine if your child has a coexisting disorder.

2. Realize that 50 to 80 percent of children with ADHD have at least one other psychological disorder. This means there is a high likelihood that your child has more than just ADHD causing his challenges.

3. Ask the professional who gave your child her diagnosis of ADHD if they also evaluated her for other disorders.

4. Know that the most common coexisting disorder is oppositional defiant disorder (ODD). The arguments, defiance, opposition, and anger that your child displays are likely due to ODD, and not solely due to symptoms of ADHD. Other coexisting disorders include learning disorder (LD), depression, anxiety, and conduct disorder.

5. Remember that learning disorders (LD) mimic the symptoms of ADHD, making it too easy to overlook the LD and blame it all on ADHD.

6. It is imperative that your child has been evaluated for LD. LD is the most overlooked disorder of childhood.

7. Do not wait until your child is in high school or college to consider the possibility of LD. The sooner it is ruled out or determined to exist, the sooner your child can get the extra help he needs.

8. Bring your child's school records to a child psychologist to screen for LD. Some children's records make it very clear there is no LD and no further action is necessary. Other children's records will indicate a potential LD, in which case formal testing is needed.

9. Testing for LD must include an IQ test and a standardized academic achievement test administered by a child clinical psychologist, educational psychologist, or neuropsychologist.

10. Do not attempt to determine your child's IQ by purchasing a test at the bookstore or online. These are not true IQ tests and have no place in a diagnostic assessment.

11. A less common coexisting disorder is Asperger's. ADHD does not mean your child is likely to have Asperger's, but having Asperger's indicates a high likelihood of having ADHD.

12. Watch for substance use or abuse in your teenager. This is a common coexisting disorder in teens with ADHD.

13. Formal testing is not usually necessary to make a diagnosis of ADHD. An experienced child psychologist can make the diagnosis based on school records, interviewing you, observing your child, and using standardized behavior questionnaires.

14. Formal testing may be needed to determine if the inattentive form of ADHD (commonly referred to as ADD) is in question. The hyperactive-impulsive form of ADHD usually does not require formal testing.

15. Understand that there is not a specific test or battery of tests that can definitively determine if your child has ADHD. Diagnosis is based on the professional's expertise and judgment, not a specific test or group of tests.

16. Do not feel shortchanged if your child's psychologist makes a rapid diagnosis. If he or she is an expert in ADHD, it is not difficult, in many cases, to know when a child has ADHD.

17. Spending more time and money on a diagnostic evaluation does not necessarily ensure a better evaluation. Spend the extra money only if the expert says he or she cannot make a determination without the extra procedures.

18. Do not spend money on any physical tests, such as MRI, PET, CT, or EEGs, looking to determine if your child has ADHD or any other mental disorder. No medical test exists to diagnose ADHD or any other psychological disorder. Anyone offering you these tests is robbing you of precious money, usually thousands of dollars, you could spend on treatment, tuition, or tutoring.

19. Make a records notebook of your child's records by category and date. You will need to have an organized record of your child on hand throughout her childhood and adolescence to share with professionals working with her.

20. Your child's records notebook should have categories for report cards, IEPs, academic achievement test scores, medical evaluations and procedures, medication, psychological evaluations and treatment, educational evaluations, and any other category of evaluation and treatment your child has had.

21. Keep a medication log in your records notebook, with the medication name, dose, date started, date ended, side effects, and responsiveness. This will be helpful to the physicians evaluating and treating your child over the years. An exact record will be far more helpful than your memory of what pill and how much you think he took when he was five and six and seven, and so on.

Tips for ACCEPTANCE

A significant amount of your success in raising your ADHD child depends on your acceptance of the reality that she has a disorder. Your acceptance will determine everything you say and do with your child. If you have a negative attitude and are skeptical of ADHD being a real disorder, or if you think your child is misbehaving on purpose or is being lazy or manipulative, you will not be able to parent your child effectively. If you have a positive attitude and accept that your child has a disorder, then you will be able to be helpful, empathic, patient, and nurturing. If you resist accepting your child for who he is, if you keep searching for a pill to make him different or a therapy to fix him, you will forever be frustrated and you will miss the joys of the uniqueness of your child. If you accept the basic facts of ADHD, you will be able to accept your child, with all her behavioral, social, and academic challenges, and you will be able to raise her in the unique way she needs to be parented.

22. Accept that your child has ADHD. Your job now is to learn the best ways to parent your special child.

23. Do not waste your time feeling guilty, wondering if you caused your child's ADHD. It is impossible to cause ADHD.

24. Recognize that while ADHD may look like a disorder of laziness, research is finding that it is a disorder of the brain's inability to regulate emotions, impulses, activity level, and attention.

25. Do not blame your child. We do not know much about the causes of ADHD; therefore, we should not be blaming the child for his symptoms that we do not understand.

26. Know that ADHD lasts at least until adolescence starts, oftentimes until or even throughout adulthood.

27. There is no cure for ADHD—end of story.

28. Focus on improving the quality of life for you, your child, and your family instead of trying to "fix it" or find a cure.

29. Stop looking for some magic solution; there is none. The solution is in your parenting.

30. The goal is to make daily life go well more often, not to make your child change.

31. Focus on what is going right, rather than what is going wrong.

32. Take a strength-based approach, rather than a deficit approach by focusing on what your child does well rather than what he does poorly.

33. If the surrounding environment is a challenge, change the environment, not the child.

34. If the current schedule is a challenge, change the schedule, not the child.

35. If you find something that works, keep doing it. Do not start looking for something else until you need to.

36. Set your expectations for your child based on how he functions now, not on how old he is.

37. Understand that ADHD children lag behind their peers on average two to three years in many areas.

38. Delete "She will never…" from your vocabulary. Most likely, she will eventually be able to do what you are expecting of her, just years later than a non-ADHD child.

39. Your child's ability to regulate himself will vary from day to day, hour to hour, so expect to have good days and bad days.

40. Remind yourself that just because your child did something well yesterday does not mean she can automatically do it well today.

41. Be exceedingly patient with your child.

42. Focus on preventing problems from happening in the first place.

43. Realize that simply teaching your child a skill is not going to make her do it. ADHD children need years of support and accommodation before a skill becomes their own.

44. Repetition is the name of the game with ADHD. To help your child learn a skill, he must repeat it over and over and over and over.

45. Offer as many supports and accommodations as necessary to make your child's daily life easier. *1000 Best Tips for ADHD* is filled with hundreds of supports and accommodations.

46. Enable your child by patiently guiding and assisting him in tasks so he eventually learns to do them on his own. Do not disable him by doing everything for him.

47. Do not believe others when they criticize accommodations and support as coddling and overprotection. ADHD children need extra support and accommodations until they are able to perform tasks and skills independently. To deny them assistance is to set a foundation for failure.

48. Believe that the support and accommodations you provide will allow your child to achieve success today so that she has the necessary skills and enough self-worth to move to the next challenge tomorrow.

49. Find solace in knowing that eventually, over the years, your child will learn how to put the supports and accommodations in place on his own and will require less of your help.

50. Find the delicate balance between helping your child flourish and thwarting her independence.

51. Help your child to swim in life by letting him experience consequences, but don't go so far as to let him drown.

52. Remember that your child will often be able to tell you what she is supposed to do, even after she has failed to do it. She may have the knowledge, but not the ability to put it into action.

53. Avoid placing too much emphasis on immediate and short-term goals, such as getting homework done and earning high grades, so that you do not miss the bigger goal of helping your child learn lifelong skills so he can function well in his adult years.

54. Balance providing assistance with letting your child learn from experience. She may have to lose recess twenty days in a row before she finally decides that she will let you help her with her homework.

55. Understand that the bad decisions your child makes can be opportunities to test out her decision-making abilities and learn from them.

56. Separate your child's successes and failures in his life from yours as a parent. His D on his essay is not your D in parenting.

57. Failures are opportunities to learn what is not working.

58. Your child's ADHD is an explanation for her behavior, but never an excuse.

59. Do not be defensive about your child's inappropriate behavior. If you are defensive, you will find that both you and your child will experience social rejection.

60. Apologize if your child acted inappropriately. Apologize appropriately and fully: "I am sorry Lewis spit at your son. He gets frustrated very easily and has not fully learned to express his anger correctly. I will have him apologize to your son. Is there anything else we can do?"

61. Do not use ADHD as an excuse. It's okay to tell others that your child has ADHD, but do not stop there. Tell them what you are doing to help your child with the problem they witnessed or experienced. "Gabby has ADHD and her impulsivity sometimes results in aggressive behavior. We have enrolled her in a kids' anger management group to help her with this." People will be more tolerant and sympathetic if they know you see the problem and are doing something about it.

62. You may think it is none of anybody's business if your child has a disorder and whether you are doing anything about it. You are correct. It really is nobody's business. However, if you want support, acceptance, and understanding from others and want your child to be included in social and family activities, a little bit of disclosure will go a long way toward achieving these goals.

63. Avoid parents who are not supportive. If disclosure has failed to result in an adult being kinder and more tolerant of your child, then that adult is best removed from the company of your child.

64. Seek out like-minded parents. You will find support, understanding, empathy, and good ideas from parents who understand the disorder and/or have a child with ADHD.

65. Avoid placing your child with adults who are rigid, impatient, and intolerant. This will only frustrate everyone involved, including your child.

66. Do not try to have adult time with your friends and relatives when you have your child with you. Schedule adult time when you do not have to be worried about your child's behavior and safety.

67. Schedule time away from your child. You deserve it and you will be more patient with your child after you have had some fun, adult time.

Tips for MEDICATION

Medication is probably the most controversial issue when it comes to raising a child with ADHD. It is never a parent's first choice to medicate his child, yet 80 percent of children with ADHD are medicated at some point. Knowing what medication can and cannot do to help your child is vital. Being informed about side effects is crucial. Formulating a philosophy about how far down the medication road you are willing to go is necessary so that you do not use medication to do what parenting is meant to. These thirty-eight tips will help you become an informed consumer about medication for ADHD.

68. Be realistic about what medication can do for your child. Medications are most effective in increasing attention, focus, and concentration and decreasing hyperactivity, impulsivity, and distractibility.

69. Know that medication will not cure your child's ADHD.

70. Become informed about the medication *before* you give it to your child.

71. Understand that all medications have risks. Learn what the risks are for your child's medication, so you can make an informed choice about your willingness to take those risks.

72. Read the information pamphlet that comes with your child's medicine, as well as the manufacturer's website. Learn all you can about the dosage, side effects, and benefits.

73. Learn what your child's medication is made of. Many parents are shocked to learn that the stimulant medication they are giving their child is made of amphetamine.

74. Reject the myth that stimulant medication has a reverse effect on children with ADHD and calms them down. Almost any person taking a low-dose amphetamine will focus better, concentrate longer, and stick to her work.

75. Understand that stimulant medication working is not proof that your child has ADHD. It will have the same effect on almost every person, even those who do not have ADHD.

76. Be sure your pediatrician is monitoring your child's cardiac health. Some children who take stimulant medication are at increased risk for cardiac events.

77. Keep a permanent notebook of all medications your child takes, with the medication name, dosage, date started, date stopped, side effects experienced, responsiveness, the reason the medication was prescribed, and the reason the medication was stopped. This will help you and your child's prescribing physician make informed medication decisions.

78. Keep all medication pamphlets in your permanent medication notebook. You may need to refer to the side effects information sometime in the future.

79. When your child starts a new medication or has any changes in dosage, keep a log of all side effects and changes. It can be difficult to remember your child's responsiveness to medications, so keep a log and bring it to your child's doctor.

80. Set realistic expectations about what medications can do. They are not magic pills or a cure in a bottle.

81. Know that medication helps with attention, concentration, hyperactivity, and impulsivity. It cannot make your child do his homework, be nice to her sister, clean her room, feed the dog, or do her book reports—you have to do that.

82. Monitor your child's mood for changes, as this can be a medication side effect.

83. Do not use medication as a stand-alone treatment. It has its best effects when used in conjunction with long-term behavior therapy.

84. Report serious side effects immediately to your doctor.

85. Schedule monthly appointments with your child's doctor. Studies show that children with ADHD who are monitored more frequently have better results than those who have traditional quarterly appointments.

86. If your child seems like a "zombie," report this to your doctor immediately. Often this indicates he is overmedicated.

87. Watch for the most common side effects, including insomnia, stomachache, decreased appetite, headache, and irritable moods. Report these to your doctor right away.

88. Acknowledge that medication is one tool that may help your child, but no child *needs* medication for ADHD.

89. Resist the temptation to judge your child's behavior on a daily basis depending on whether he took his medication. We all have good days and bad days, and so do children who take ADHD medications.

90. Resist pressure from your child's teacher to medicate your child. It is your choice, and no school can force you to medicate your child.

91. Avoid repeatedly changing medications, looking for the perfect pill. Medicated children will continue to have ADHD symptoms, just at a lower intensity and frequency.

92. Understand that the majority of behavior problems children with ADHD have cannot be medicated away. Medication will not stop lying, teasing, messy rooms, low self-esteem, poor social skills, obsession with video games, etc.

93. If your child's personality changes when she is medicated, inform your doctor, as this should not happen.

94. Medication is a lot of trial and error. The first prescription is rarely the right medication at the right dose at the right time. Decide how much experimenting you are willing to put your child through.

95. Tics can start after stimulant medications and warrant an immediate call to your doctor.

96. Do not go along with any doctor who tells you tics are an acceptable side effect. There is a high likelihood they will become permanent.

97. Be very cautious when your child's doctor wants to use another medication to deal with a side effect of the first medication.

98. Ask yourself why you are medicating your child. Answers such as "she needs it" or "she cannot function without it" are not reality based. No child with ADHD needs stimulant medication. Your child is most likely functioning, just not as well as you would like.

99. Never ask "Did you take your medicine?" in the same conversation about a problem behavior. This says to your child that the medicine determines whether he can behave.

100. Do not blame or thank the medicine. The medicine is a tool to help your child tap into self-control that is harder to tap into unmedicated, but it is not what makes her have self-control or lose self-control.

101. Always maintain control over your child's medication, regardless of his age. Many high school students take extra pills and give or sell them to their peers.

102. Educate your high school– or college-age child that selling and giving away her medication is a crime. Many colleges are eager to stop this crime and are taking action to prosecute.

103. Ask yourself what you would do if medication was not an option for your child. You would have to learn the skills necessary to create an environment where your child can flourish and succeed despite her symptoms.

104. Consider medication during vacation time. Parents of children who take medications for attention issues to help with schoolwork and homework sometimes choose to allow a break from medication during vacations. Many parents of children with behavior problems of hyperactivity and impulsivity choose to have their child medicated even during vacation periods. Discuss your options with your child's prescribing physician.

105. Consider vacation time an opportunity for your child to experience what it is like to be himself without medication. Discuss this with his prescribing physician.

Common ADHD Behavior

Tips for
BETTER BEHAVIOR

Children with ADHD have behavior problems in many areas of life; it is simply the nature of the disorder. Children with ADHD do not mean to misbehave; they just forget to do what they know is right. They may hear what you say, but immediately forget it. They may remember what you said, but something distracted them and grabbed their attention. They may start the task you ask but have no idea how to go about the steps to completing it. These symptoms of ADHD mean you have to be on your best parenting behavior at all times. Relax a little, and your child's behavior suffers. These eighteen tips for behavior will ensure that you have a sound foundation for managing your child's behavior.

106. Expect behavior problems to happen every day, and then do not be surprised and angry when they do.

107. Prevention is your first parenting tool. Any problem that can be prevented is a problem that does not have to be solved. If your child forgets her lunch box almost every day, instead of nagging, punishing, or removing privileges, just put her lunch in her backpack for her. Do not worry; eventually she will remember to take her own lunch.

108. Be wise and supervise. Children with ADHD need almost constant supervision; otherwise, they find themselves in frequent problematic or dangerous situations.

109. Know what your child is doing at all times. ADHD children have very poor judgment and they do not anticipate danger or problems, so you have to anticipate for them.

110. When your child is not in the same room with you, set your cell phone alarm to go off every fifteen minutes to remind you to check on him.

111. Make a rule notebook where you and your child write the rules one by one. Make a page for each category of behavior, including rules for bedtime, use of computer and other electronic devices, aggression, chores, and homework. Include what happens if the rule is followed and what happens if the rule is broken.

112. Limit the number of rules you have to the ones you know you will reinforce; otherwise, you are teaching your child that you have many rules, but she only has to follow a few of them.

113. Evenly enforce all the rules you make; otherwise, you teach your child to gamble on whether he will get in trouble for breaking a rule.

114. Rule-breaking must be followed by some type of consequence, even if it is just a disapproving comment or a calm talk about why the behavior was wrong. Ignoring rule-breaking sends the message that it is acceptable to break some of the rules some of the time.

115. If you are not going to enforce a rule because you are too tired, too busy, or for any other reason, be honest with yourself and limit the number of rules you have to enforce. No parent can enforce every rule, so focus on those that are most important and let the others go until you know you can enforce them.

116. Modify your rules as needed. ADHD children change rapidly, so the rules need to keep pace.

117. Ignore minor annoying but non-rule-breaking behaviors. Humming, fidgeting, pencil tapping, and other behaviors are best ignored. You won't be able to stop them anyway, so ignore as much as you can.

118. Follow the rules of society and the law. Your actions are louder than your words. Act in proper ways so your child will do the same.

119. Keep a daily log or chart of the behaviors your child is working on. It is difficult to tell if changes in your parenting are resulting in changes in your child's behavior unless you keep accurate data. Relying on your memory and your feelings about how your child is doing is a sure way to fail at behavior management.

120. Charting your child's behavior will help you look for patterns of when things are going right and when they are going wrong. Chart which tip you are using, what time and where the tip was used, who was involved, and how your child responded. Make note of any deviations you made in using the tip.

121. When your child finds success in a behavior, let him own that success by not adding more requirements too soon. Let a few weeks go by before you raise your expectations.

122. Increase expectations in small increments. Do not be so eager to get your child to meet your expectations that you rob her of feeling good about her progress and make her feel that she can never make you happy.

123. Try to understand why a particular problem behavior keeps happening over and over. A functional behavioral analysis looks at the purpose of a behavior to discover what can be done to change it. Create a daily log of when, where, and how a problem behavior takes place and what happens afterward. After a few days to a few weeks, you may be able to determine why the behavior occurs. If your son has a tantrum every night at bedtime, what is the result of the tantrum? What does he get by having a tantrum that he would not get if he simply went to bed? It may be as simple as staying awake fifteen minutes longer; if so, change his bedtime so he can stay up fifteen minutes later and maybe the tantrums will stop. If he gets you to lie down with him by having a tantrum, try lying down with him right away and see if he skips the tantrum.

Tips for ANGER

Difficulties with anger are a common occurrence with ADHD. It is easy to get entangled in power struggles with your child, especially if you believe that her anger is a manipulative attempt to get her own way. While anger outbursts and tantrums can surely look manipulative, we have recent research that suggests that children and teens with ADHD have delayed brain development in the limbic system, the area of the brain where emotions are thought to originate. As a result of immature brain development, you are likely to see immature emotional reactions. You may also see explosive anger, aggression, and tantrums due to what researchers are theorizing to be poor development of the frontal lobe, the part of the brain that allows us to stop ourselves from acting upon our impulses. Children with ADHD have an anger switch that is too easy to turn on and quite difficult to turn off. Through no fault of their own, they overreact to upset and have great difficulty controlling their feelings and impulses to act out their anger. Understanding that anger outbursts are not purposeful can help you to stay calm and use tips that will allow your child to manage his anger in appropriate ways.

124. Prevention is your first tool in helping your child manage her anger. Structure your life and household so that, as much as possible, upsets are prevented.

125. ADHD children can escalate very rapidly in their anger from mild frustration to rageful outbursts in a matter of seconds. Stay calm and remind yourself that this is your child's anger and you do not have to be angry just because he is.

126. Monitor your child closely for signs that she is on the brink of an anger outburst so you can defuse the situation and prevent it.

127. Try to recognize the anger as soon as it begins to surface. Use your child's anger as a signal that you need to take a few deep breaths before you respond. This will give you time to think about a rational and calm response.

128. Your anger and your child's anger are frequently intertwined. If you get angry, you must expect that your child will surely get angry too.

129. Children with ADHD are incredibly sensitive to your anger. Monitor your voice tone and volume so that your child can listen to your words rather than your anger.

130. If you feel yourself on the brink of losing control over your words or actions, give yourself a time out and come back to deal with your child when you are calm.

131. If you feel too angry to talk with your child in a manner that helps him realize his misdeeds, try to delay your talk until you can be a helper instead of a punisher.

132. Being able to talk about your parenting frustrations with another adult will help you discharge your anger in healthy ways and decrease the chance that you will take it out on your child.

133. Learning how to be angry in healthy ways does not come naturally to anyone. You must teach your child specific anger-management skills.

134. Take inventory of your anger management skills. What are you doing when you are angry that you see your child mimicking?

135. Learn a variety of anger management techniques so you are in control of your anger.

136. When you are angry, tell your child which skills you are using to calm yourself down. "I am so upset right now I can't talk nicely, so I am going to take some deep breaths until I can think of nice words to use." "I am really angry right now, so I am going to take a hot bath and calm down."

137. Let your child know that everyone feels angry and it is a normal part of life.

138. Be sure your child knows that anger is something that we have to experience and not run away from. Anger has to come out and not be held in.

139. Teach your child to take three deep breaths when she is angry. Repeat as necessary until she is able to talk and behave in a controlled fashion.

140. Encourage your child to work out his anger physically by shooting hoops, running, jumping rope, throwing mud balls, hitting his pillow, etc.

141. Show your child how to use writing or typing as a way to express her angry thoughts and feelings. Be sure to remind her not to send the letter to anyone so no one gets their feelings hurt.

142. Start an anger diary for you and your child to pass back and forth. You can take turns writing to one another what you are angry about and which solutions you think might solve the situation.

143. Have your child try counting out loud backward when he is angry. This interrupts angry thoughts and requires mental effort that results in a decrease in anger.

144. Actively listen to your child when he is upset. Be patient and let him talk and vent his frustration. Active listening means truly listening, not interrupting or thinking about what you are going to say. You will learn why he is upset if you listen more and talk less.

145. Use reflection when your child verbalizes her anger. If she screams "You are so unfair!" resist the temptation to explain why you are fair or give the typical "Life isn't always fair" retort. Instead, reflect back to her what she said by restating or rephrasing, "You are mad because I won't let you have a slumber party." This lets her know you actually heard what she is upset about.

146. Use empathy to let your child know that you understand what he is feeling. An empathic statement lets your child know that you can see why he is feeling the way he is. It does not mean you necessarily agree with his emotions, but you are saying "I can understand why you feel so mad right now."

147. Use resolution to solve the problem that made your child mad. After you have actively listened, reflected, and validated, you can then invite your child to suggest a resolution. A genuine desire for what she sees as a solution lets her know that you want to work with her to solve the situation and prevent it from recurring. A good starting question is: "What do you think we can do so that this does not happen again?"

148. When your child is offering a solution to a problem that made him mad, regardless of how improbable the suggestion might be, listen to it and respond with a positive attitude that encourages him to continue to work with you. "So you would like to be in charge of your backpack and not have me go into it. That is one option we can talk about."

149. Resist the urge to tell her why her solution would never work, how she failed at it last time she tried it, or that she is incapable of keeping this agreement. You want her to learn how to solve problems and think of solutions. Active listening and validating her suggestion as one option lets her know that you are open to her ideas rather than just telling her what to do.

150. Offer your solution as another option and give your reasoning behind it. "I was thinking that I could check your backpack every other day instead of daily. This way, we would be trying out your solution of letting you be in charge of your backpack three days each week, and I would only check it two days. You and I both want you to succeed and not fall behind in homework. I fear that if we go from me checking it daily to not checking it at all, you risk falling behind very quickly. What do you think about us agreeing to two days each week and we will see how it goes? We can change it to less often if it is going well or more often if we find that you do better when I help you."

151. When you use a resolution approach, your child's anger will slowly decrease and he will learn that if he is angry, he does not have to escalate to get your attention, be heard by you, or get you to agree to other options.

Tips for FIDGETING

Inability to sit still is a hallmark symptom of ADHD. Wiggling, fidgeting, and constantly moving in a seat can cause distraction and frequent opportunities for reprimands. We do not know why children with ADHD have such a strong need to move. Some researchers hypothesize that they have a need to seek physical sensation. Others guess that it is the inability of the frontal lobe of the brain to put the brake pedal on movement. Still others think it may be due to a need to fight boredom and keep the brain stimulated. Whatever the cause, we have not found a way to keep it under control. While medication can help, it does not cure fidgeting and only helps during the times when the medication is active in the system. The best approach to date is to simply understand that fidgeting is a part of the disorder that we cannot stop, and instead we need to find ways to work around it and not let it interfere with daily life.

152.   Understand that fidgeting is not bad. It can be annoying, yes, but it's not bad.

153. Know that some research suggests that children may actually concentrate better if they are moving.

154. Accept that fidgeting does not need to be stopped. It does not need to be medicated away. Nothing awful will happen if you let your child fidget.

155. Allow your child to fidget. You won't be able to stop it, so do your best to ignore it whenever possible.

156. Understand that trying to get your child to stop fidgeting will be an endless, impossible quest. He may stop for a moment, but he will soon be at it again. How much time do you want to devote to trying to stop something that cannot be stopped?

157. Before you direct your child to stop fidgeting, ask yourself if it is really necessary that he stop. What will happen if you just let him fidget away to his heart's content?

158. Try not to be annoyed by your child's fidgeting. If left alone, fidgeting is really not much of a problem for the child. The biggest problem is that it annoys adults.

159. Monitor your child's fidgeting and your reaction to it.

Do the problems with her fidgeting start when you try to get her to stop? If so, quit directing her to stop and just let her fidget.

160. Provide your child with a fidget object. Just like many adults like to hold a pen while they read, work, and talk, children like to hold something in their hands as well.

161. Stress balls allow your child to squeeze an object quietly and satisfy his urge to seek physical stimulation.

162. Rubber bracelets, the kind that are popular with many charities, are good, durable fidget objects that won't disturb anyone.

163. Be aware that fidgeting can be soothing and some children may use repetitive, rhythmic movement as a means to keep calm.

164. Forget the myth that children cannot learn if they are moving. This is simply not true. In fact, movement is increasingly being found to enhance learning.

165. Fidgeting, wiggling, tapping feet, and even chewing gum have been found to increase concentration.

166. Large exercise balls can help wiggling children sit longer. They can wiggle and squirm without leaving their seat or distracting anyone.

167. Sitting in a beanbag chair can decrease squirming and wiggling and the desire to get out of one's seat.

168. Pacing while thinking, reciting, or answering questions can help some children think better.

169. Jumping rope or bouncing a ball while reciting short bits of information can increase your child's ability to memorize things like spelling words or multiplication tables.

170. Standing up at a desk can help concentration, focus, and perseverance in tasks for some children.

171. Rocking chairs provide rhythmic movement that can help concentration.

172. Doodling can decrease fidgeting and squirming.

173. Talk with your child's teacher about ignoring fidgeting so that your child is not frequently reprimanded or pointed out in class as being a problem.

174. Ask the teacher's permission for your child to have a fidget object on his desk.

175. Provide a fidget object for your child in situations where she is likely to fidget. The top situations where fidgeting will occur include at school, at religious services, at restaurants, and while doing homework.

Tips for FOCUSING

Trouble focusing is one of the symptoms required to be diagnosed with ADHD. Difficulty focusing accompanies poor concentration, trouble sticking to a task, and problems ignoring distractions. Children with ADHD have trouble focusing in class, during homework, when their parents are talking to them, and anytime they are doing an undesirable activity. Yet, put them in front of the television, computer, or video game and suddenly they have perfect focus that can last for hours. This is one of the most frustrating quandaries for parents. Researchers do not understand why this is but suggest that something in the brains of children with ADHD requires a high level of reward and stimulation to hold their attention. Boring tasks make their brains drowsy, sluggish, and distractible. We can't make their brains different, but we can use these thirteen tips to help them focus more often and for longer periods of time.

176. Use earplugs or certain sounds (noise machines or soft, mellow music with a repetitive, rhythmic beat and no lyrics) to block out distracting background noises to encourage concentration in children.

177. Realize that having to focus feels like torture for many children with ADHD. Some children would rather sit in time-out for two hours than do fifteen minutes of work that requires focusing. It takes so much mental effort to focus that it is miserable to them.

178. Knowing how much your child likely dreads having to focus on something he finds boring and difficult, you must be able to make it exciting, or at least make the reward for completing it exciting.

179. A timer set to ring every five minutes during homework will remind your child to focus.

180. Use gentle physical cues to refocus your child on his work. A tap of your pencil on his paper or a touch on his shoulder can be used as signals to get back to work.

181. Focusing for short periods of time with short rest breaks can ease the stress of homework. Try fifteen minutes of work with one-minute breaks as a starting point and alter as needed.

182. Use a place-marker to help your child keep focused on where she is supposed to be looking in her book or on her paper.

183. Have your child do an action when he is studying, such as using a highlighter, making index cards, underlining key words, or telling you what he just read. Using action-oriented study skills increases focus.

184. Resign yourself to sitting with your child while she does her homework so that you can keep her on task.

185. Reduce distractions and create a quiet environment for your child to work. This means TV is off, siblings are quiet, music is off or low.

186. Select a study space that has very few visual distractions. Close the blinds, have the dog lay down or go in another room, and remove anything from the table that is not homework-related.

187. Make a reading window out of a file folder. Cut out a rectangle big enough to allow two to three lines of text and use the rest of the file folder to cover the other text on the page. This will help cut out visual distractions.

188. A metronome has been found to increase concentration in some children as it gives a quiet, rhythmic sound.

Tips for
FORGETFULNESS

Forgetfulness is another hallmark symptom of ADHD. It disrupts daily life multiple times each day. Your child may be on the way to the bathroom to brush his teeth but forget halfway there where he is going and why he is supposed to go there. While this looks like defiance, it is more likely due to forgetfulness. We do not know what is going awry in their brains' memory functioning, but children with ADHD have a very hard time holding thoughts in their minds. What they hear in their immediate memory somehow gets lost and never makes it to short-term memory. Through no fault of their own, things go in one ear and out the other. These thirty-four tips will help your child get through his day with helpful ways that work with his forgetfulness.

189. Realize that children with ADHD truly have trouble remembering what they are supposed to do, how to do it, when to do it, and why they have to do it.

190. Try to remind yourself that forgetfulness is a symptom of ADHD and not purposeful noncompliance. Noncompliance is an outright, purposeful refusal that looks very different from forgetfulness.

191. You will be more patient when you understand that children with ADHD may have their routines, tasks, and rules memorized in their long-term memory, but something in the way their brains function does not allow them to access those long-term memories for immediate use. They need help pulling those long-term memories out of storage so they can be used in present time.

192. Memorize the term "working memory." This is the part of our memory that we use when we are listening and trying to store in our minds what we are hearing.

193. Know that children with ADHD have very poor working memory. They can only hold tiny bits of information in their working memory.

194. Give only one directive or verbal instruction at a time. Do not give another one until the first one has been completed.

195. If you give multiple directives or instructions, your child may forget all of them and make it appear that he is being noncompliant.

196. If you believe your child is often noncompliant, pay attention to how you are giving her directives. Watch to see if you are giving too many directives and too much information at one time.

197. When you give a directive or instruction, ask your child to repeat it back to you. This ensures she heard it correctly and helps her memorize the directive by saying it aloud and hearing herself say it.

198. Teach your child to use self-talk, which is saying the directive over and over aloud to herself. This will increase her ability to remember what she is supposed to be doing.

199. Use visual cues as often as you can. Children with ADHD do far better remembering things when they have visual cues. Remember this mantra: "Tell me, and I forget. Show me, and I remember."

200. Make task cards out of index cards to help your child complete his tasks. Give your child a card with one task on it and tell him to bring it back when he has finished the task. Then give him the next task card.

201. Task cards are simple phrases that state only the task to be done: "Brush your teeth," "Put your pajamas on," and "Put your backpack by the front door" are some examples.

202. Task cards with a picture of the task are good to use, as they provide visual cues, which are easier to follow than written cues. Select age-appropriate pictures and change them as your child matures.

203. After your child completes one task, be sure to praise her.

204. If your child is on a token economy/point program to earn rewards and privileges, give him his tokens/points before assigning the next task.

205. Make individual task cards for tasks you know your child forgets how to do. Type or write out step-by-step instructions.

206. Make a to-do list each day for your child to use to tell him what he needs to do and in what order.

207. Since many children's schedules are the same from day to day, you can make the to-do lists on your computer and modify them as necessary.

208. To-do lists for young children work well when there is a picture showing each task. You can cut pictures from a magazine, get them from the Internet, or use a photo of your child doing the task.

209. Make the to-do list age-appropriate. Young children will enjoy a large poster board with colorful pictures and letters; teens will want a simple typed list on regular paper.

210. Written instructions are easier for children with ADHD to follow than those given orally. It is easy for a child with ADHD to forget what he just heard. Reading it again helps refresh his memory.

211. Have your child cross off each task as it is done. This gives her a sense of control over herself and a feeling of independence and accomplishment when she crosses off each task.

212. Instead of nagging, tell your child, "Go check your to-do list. If you can't figure it out, then come ask me what to do next."

213. Make a daily to-do list for yourself and let your child see you using it. He will be more likely to use his list if he sees that you use one too.

214. To help your child decrease repeated breaking of the same rules, post a rule chart where it can easily be seen. Many teachers post rule charts in their classrooms, and this strategy can work in the home too.

215. Technology is your friend in the world of forgetfulness. When age-appropriate, help your child use her cell phone to set the alarm to go off for tasks.

216. A digital watch with an alarm can be used for task reminders for children who are not old enough for a cell phone.

217. Empathize with your child's forgetfulness by realizing we all have a bit of trouble with memory at times.

218. Put the cell phone to good use by texting your child when she has a task to do. Ask her to text you back when she has finished it.

219. Have your child use his cell phone to email or text himself his homework assignments. Be sure he has permission to do this from his teacher.

220. Have your child use the voice memo feature on her cell phone to record homework assignments. Be sure she has permission to do this from her teacher.

221. Packing checklists will prevent forgetfulness. Make checklists for packing lunches, backpacks, sports equipment, etc. Keep these lists on your computer and print as necessary.

222. Laminate to-do and packing checklists that your child uses frequently. An erasable grease pencil can be used to check off items.

Tips for
INTERRUPTING

Talking too much, talking over others, butting into conversations, blurting out answers in class: all symptoms of ADHD. All are symptoms of impulsivity that are very difficult for ADHD children to control and parents to manage. Children with ADHD seem to have no stop sign between thought and speaking. Part of this seems due to the brain's poor development in inhibition where they cannot stop themselves and feel that they *must* say what they are thinking. Another part seems due to poor working memory where those with ADHD cannot hold a thought in their minds for even a few seconds before they forget what they wanted to say. This leads to great frustration and has the unfortunate result of the child concluding that interrupting is the only way he can get his thoughts voiced. Add a little bit of emotional immaturity and self-centeredness, where the child believes what he has to say is so important that it would be a tragedy if he were to forget it because he had to wait, and you have a child who frequently interrupts.

223. Interrupting is part of the impulsivity of ADHD. Understanding that it is a chronic symptom can help you be more patient with your child.

224. Expect that your child will have problems with interrupting for years beyond what you would anticipate. Interrupting can be one of the most resistant symptoms, and many adults with ADHD still struggle with trying to refrain from interrupting.

225. Create a signal between you and your child that she can use when she wants to tell you something when you are talking to someone else. Acknowledge her signal by nodding your head or giving the signal back; otherwise, she most likely will keep interrupting you.

226. Teach your child to gently touch you once on the arm to let you know he wants to talk. You can touch back to acknowledge his request and keep your hand on him to keep him calm and aware that you have not forgotten that he wants to talk.

227. Your child will respond better to your teaching him not to interrupt if you do not make him wait for long before responding. Since children with ADHD are very poor at estimating time, waiting a few seconds can seem like minutes to them. The longer he feels he is waiting, the more impatient and frustrated he will become. As he improves with waiting for a few seconds, you can very slowly extend how long you make him wait.

228. Use any object to pass between you and your child when having a conversation. Only the person holding the object can talk. Many children respond well to a toy microphone.

229. Praise your child when she refrains from interrupting. Be specific in your praise: "I really liked it when you stood near me and waited for me to finish my sentence before you started talking."

230. Reward your child with points/tokens when he demonstrates that he is not interrupting. Immediately tell him: "I am going to give you five bonus points because you did such a good job waiting your turn to speak."

231. Teach your child that it is OK to interrupt you when there is an emergency. Define for her what an emergency is, such as fire, someone hurt, or the dog escaping from the yard.

232. Prompt your child to say "Excuse me" when he wants to interrupt.

233. Expect your child to say "Excuse me" and then continue without pausing to tell you what she wants to say. Teach her that "Excuse me" does not mean she can keep talking; she needs to wait until you tell her it is okay to talk.

Tips for a Happy Home

Tips for CHORES

Few children like to do chores. ADHD children are particularly resistant to engaging in any task that does not provide excitement and fun. Arguments over chores are a common occurrence in ADHD households, but this does not have to be the case. Understanding that children with ADHD have limited attention, a low tolerance for boredom, and a high drive for rewards will provide you with the perfect formula for getting chores completed. Chores have to be short, done one at a time, and followed by an immediate reward. Follow these forty tips and you will be certain to find chore time easier.

234. Most children dislike chores, so drop any expectations that your child will do them without grumbling.

235. Your child will be more compliant with chores if she earns tokens/points for completing them. They can later be traded in for privileges and rewards.

236. Rewarding your child for completing chores is a way to teach him that work leads to reward, which is, after all, how our society is set up: go to work, get a paycheck, trade that paycheck in for rewards. Rewarding a child for completing chores is not bribing him; it is rewarding him, just like your employer rewards you with a paycheck.

237. Use a chart that lists the chores, and assign a token/point value to each chore.

238. For younger children, make charts using pictures of the chore instead of words.

239. Hang the chart where your child can easily see it so he can frequently look at his success.

240. Immediately after one chore is done, have your child write the points on her chart so she experiences the immediate reward and the sense of self-satisfaction. Younger children can put on stars, happy faces, or stickers instead of writing points.

241. Do not delay putting points on the chart. ADHD children quickly lose motivation if they do not get instant gratification for their work.

242. Drop the expectation that your child should learn to do chores because he is part of the family and should want to contribute. Instead, create a family atmosphere where those who contribute to the family get rewarded, and those who do not contribute do not get rewarded.

243. You do not have to spend money on rewards for your child completing chores. Tokens/points that can be traded in for privileges such as computer or TV time, going to the park, and edible treats work very well.

244. Allow your child to access her earned privileges only after her chores are done. Do not buy into the famous line, "I will do it later."

245. Teach your child to help, beginning in the toddler years. Picking up toys will be the first task your child will learn. Intense defiance when it is time to pick up toys is often one of the first signs of ADHD. Parents who give in to this first battle are setting the pattern for tantrums, resulting in your child escaping from the task. Toddlers and young children, of course, need your help. For a toddler who outright refuses to clean up, gently place your hand over his hand and pleasantly physically guide him to pick up the toy and put it away. Repeat until he picks up toys without your hand on his. This is not a punishment, but a way for you to help him. Praise the very second he complies.

246. Make chores age-appropriate. A toddler picks up her toys with your help, a five-year-old puts her clothes in the hamper while you supervise, a seven-year-old helps set the table under your direction, a nine-year-old takes out the trash, etc.

247. Use colored index cards to write one chore per card so your child can use them as a visual aid.

248. Laminate the chore cards so you can use them over and over. In place of a laminator, a sandwich bag or plastic wrap will keep the card intact for many uses.

249. Write only one chore per card so your child is focused on the one chore and not overwhelmed by a list of chores.

250. Glue a photo of the chore onto the card and write step-by-step instructions. This provides a visual aid for your child to refer to so he does not have to rely on his memory.

251. Be very specific in the instructions. You cannot write "clean your bedroom" on a card and expect it to be done.

Instead, select one specific task that is part of cleaning a bedroom and give that one card to your child to complete. Your clean bedroom cards can be broken down into separate cards with one task per card: "Put all toys in your toy basket," "Put all dirty clothes in your clothes hamper," "Put all shoes on your closet floor," etc. Each task is on its own card, given out one at a time.

252. When it is chore time, give your child one chore card at a time and have her return it to you when the chore is complete. Do not give more than one chore card at a time, as it is too overwhelming for a child with ADHD to think about all the chores that must be completed.

253. After your child returns the chore card, have him show you the completed chore. Praise and give him points for completion before giving him the next chore card.

254. Praise effort even if your child has not yet achieved perfect success in her task.

255. Praise small steps toward progress. Psychologists call this "successive approximations." Break the chore into tiny steps and praise the smallest success, then slowly increase your requirements. For example, you would not expect your child to make the bed perfectly. At age five, you might expect her to place the pillow at the head of the bed; at age six, she can pull the bedspread up; at age seven, she can pull the sheets and blanket up; etc.

256. Do chores together. The old phrase "misery loves company" is really true when we are doing tasks we would prefer to skip. Having someone alongside you makes it easier. Your child will cooperate more if you are doing a task with him, or at least doing another task while he does his.

257. Show your child how to do the task, have her do it, and praise her. Children with ADHD learn better visually than verbally. Showing is better than telling.

258. Do not expect your child to successfully complete chores on his own. Your direction will be needed.

259. Drop any expectation that your child will do her chores without being told. It just won't happen. You must prompt her to do them and supervise to ensure they are done.

260. Set a time to do chores, rather than leaving them for whenever time allows.

261.   Remind your child ahead of time that chores will be done today. Give frequent countdown reminders in time periods of one hour, thirty minutes, ten minutes, and five minutes.

262.   Chores first, playtime second. Do not give in to begging, pleading, or promising to do it later.

263.   Use "When you…then you may…" phrases, such as "When you empty the dishwasher, then you may go outside and play."

264.   Forget the nagging. Make a written contact for chores that describes what chores are to be done, when they are to be done, and what rewards will be earned. If chores are not done, rewards are not given. Place this contract in your rule notebook, or add it to your posted list of rules.

265.   Reminders to do chores are not the same as nagging. Nagging is repeated and escalating. Reminders are planned and timed appropriately before the chore is expected to be done.

266.   Do not get into a battle over chores. Chores not done do not earn rewards.

267. If your child refuses to do certain chores that must be done and cannot be delayed, such as cleaning his room when company is coming over, you can do the chore and remove the equivalent tokens/points from his bank or money from his allowance to pay yourself for having done the chore. This is the rare time that tokens or points can be removed for noncompliance.

268. Keep the number of chores limited to one or two easy chores per day, or less. ADHD children are easily overwhelmed, and too many chores for some can be the tipping point into meltdowns.

269. Carefully choose which chores you will insist on and which ones are not worth it. Battles over cleaning the bedroom might be better dropped so that your child has time to do more important tasks, such as homework.

270. Choose chores based upon how your child functions in daily life, rather than based on her age. If your child struggles to get through basic tasks such as getting out of bed, getting dressed for school, getting homework done, etc., she is probably not ready to do anything more than very simple, quick chores, such as hanging up her bath towel and putting clothes in the hamper.

271. Start with chores that you are certain your child can successfully complete. This will create a positive experience of what it is like to do chores.

272. Let your child help out whenever he asks or shows interest. Many children are eager to vacuum because they like to push a loud machine around. Even though he won't do it perfectly, let him do it anyway. You can always touch it up later.

273. To encourage helping with the dishes, let your child help with the cooking and baking. She will be more willing to do the boring task if she is able to do the fun task first.

Tips for EATING

The biggest problems with eating for children with ADHD fall under the categories of picky eating and lack of appetite. Two of the most common side effects of stimulant medication are stomachaches and loss of appetite. A more flexible attitude about food and a bit of cleverness can help you get around these obstacles and ensure your child is consuming enough calories and nutrients. Try these twenty tips to improve your child's eating.

274. Do not expect eliminating sugar and food additives to make your child less active and impulsive. Unfortunately, it is the rare child who has behavior problems simply because of what he eats.

275. If you try an elimination diet, you must do it systematically. Keep a detailed log of your child's behavior for two weeks. Eliminate one food for two weeks and continue to keep a log of behavior. Reintroduce the eliminated food for two weeks while logging behavior. This detailed analysis may tell you if that one food has any impact on your child's functioning. Repeat this procedure food by food.

276. Eliminating foods can be an enticing way to go because it offers parents a real sense of control. However, since most children do not have problems due to food, the only thing parents are controlling is their grocery shopping. Food offers little in the way of getting your child to do her homework, go to bed on time, complete her chores, be nice to her sister, etc.

277. There is some recent research on a small group of children that found eliminating artificial additives and preservatives had modest effects on behavior. There is no harm in trying to eliminate certain unnatural substances. Just keep a realistic perspective and do not expect dramatic changes. Even if there are no behavior changes, you will be providing your child with a healthier diet that is better for his body.

278. Keep an eating log when your child starts a medication or changes the dosage or type of medicine to determine if the medicine is affecting your child's appetite. Log height, weight, and what, when, and how much she eats. Some children adapt to the appetite suppressant side effects in a few weeks and return to their normal eating habits. Others never adapt and continue to have little desire to eat when taking medication. Be sure to show your eating log to your prescribing physician.

279. Feed your child before or while she takes her medication to ensure she gets enough calories before the medication kicks in and decreases her appetite.

280. Feed your child whenever he is hungry if he is taking stimulant medication. The normal rules of not allowing eating in between or after meals have to be forgotten when your child is taking stimulant medications. When the medication wears off, appetite often increases, causing your child to be hungry at times that do not coincide with normal meals.

281. Be flexible about the variety of foods you have available for your child if she is taking medication. Eating something, even if not the most nutritious food, is better than your child not taking in any calories.

282. Try fruit and energy bars for a tasty snack packed with nutrients.

283. Smoothies are an easy way to pack in a lot of calories, and adding yogurt or ice cream to smoothies makes them creamy, tasty, and calorie-dense.

284. Blending frozen fruit into a smoothie adds bulk to fill up the tummy and provides good nutrients. A scoop of protein powder in a smoothie adds the one essential food group your child is most likely to resist.

285. Pack extra calories and nutrition in muffins, cakes, and pancakes by adding protein powder.

286. Do not use the removal of food as a punishment, especially if your child is on medication.

287. Six smaller meals per day are recommended for children with ADHD rather than the old school of thought of three large meals.

288. Be sure your child has breakfast every day, as it truly is important to give him energy to fuel his brain during school. Go beyond traditional breakfast foods and let your child eat calorie-dense foods that might otherwise be lunch or dinner options.

289. Be flexible about breakfast. Whoever said that breakfast must be limited to cereal, eggs, pancakes, and waffles? Pizza, pasta, and burritos, for example, may be more attractive and offer needed calories and nutrition.

290. Have portable breakfasts packed and ready to grab and eat en route to school. Many children with ADHD move too slowly in the morning to have enough time for a sit-down breakfast. Never deny your child breakfast because she was too slow getting ready and ran out of time.

291. Monitor your child's lunch box for what comes back home on a regular basis. Send foods you know he will eat.

292. Ask your child if she eats what you pack for lunch or if she trades or throws it out. Assure her she is not in trouble and that you only want to send her with food she will eat.

293. Remember that sugar is not evil. Post-meal sweet treats can be powerful motivators for children to clean their plates.

Tips for ORGANIZATION

Children with ADHD are messy, easily lose their belongings, and have little motivation to be organized and keep track of their items. Repeated loss of jackets, backpacks, lunch boxes, homework, school notes, papers, projects, and textbooks can be expected. Organization is a frontal lobe skill that is typically poorly developed in children with ADHD and one they have little interest is mastering. Expect that you will have to supply this frontal lobe skill for your child for years longer than you think should be necessary. Poor organization is one of the most resistant symptoms of ADHD, and it can often linger well on into adult years. Taking charge of organizing your child's belongings, school work, homework, sports, and extracurricular activities will save many arguments and tears. Fortunately, there are many modern tools that make organization easier for you and your child. Try some of these forty-two tips to see which best suits your lifestyle.

294. Organize your household and keep it that way.

Children with ADHD function better in neat, organized, and structured environments.

295. Don't expect your child to know how to organize his room, backpack, or belongings. Set up the structure for him by labeling drawers, shelves, and containers in his room.

296. Once you have a room that is highly organized and labeled for your child, expect that, for many years, you will still have to manage keeping things where they belong.

297. To-do lists are the most useful organization tool for families living with ADHD. Do not expect or pressure yourself or your child to remember all the things you have to do.

298. Use computer software for notes to put to-do tasks on your child's computer desktop. She can delete them when the task is done and email you a note that she completed the task.

299. Use a computer calendar to schedule repetitive activities, such as extracurricular events, and color-code them for easy visual cues for you and your child to see.

300. Use colorful sticky notes or paper for reminders and tape them where your child will see them, such as on a bathroom mirror, closet door, or cell phone.

301. Change the color and style of your sticky notes frequently, as your child will get used to seeing them and they will no longer be novel or catch his attention.

302. Use a large dry-erase board to create a weekly calendar to hang on the wall where your child can easily see what is scheduled for the week.

303. Color-coordinate activities on the calendar: green for sports, blue for homework, yellow for doctor's appointments, etc.

304. Post all upcoming events on a calendar for your child to see.

305. Warn your child ahead of time of upcoming changes to the ordinary routine.

306. Motivate your child to do a twice-annual bedroom cleaning by having a garage sale and letting her keep the money for the items she sells from her room.

307. Have your child empty her backpack every day and repack things neatly when her homework is done.

308. Color-code your child's school materials. Each subject is assigned a color and all materials for that subject are that color. This makes it easy to find all the necessary items for each subject. Textbooks, notebooks, flash cards, and highlighters should all be the same color for one subject. Textbooks can be wrapped in a colored book cover or your child can decorate a plain cover with colored paper and markers.

309. Provide color-coded stacking bins for your child's returned homework, tests, and projects. Use one bin per subject for easy retrieval when it is time to study for tests.

310. Place a small basket in your child's homework area to put in papers that he no longer needs to carry in his backpack but are not appropriate for throwing away.

311. Use color-coded plastic folders with Velcro fasteners for each subject to keep homework and school papers in so they won't fall out.

312. Use one plastic folder with a Velcro fastener labeled "To Be Turned In" to put your child's homework and notes to be signed in. This will save homework from getting lost between home and the classroom.

313. For children who have a difficult time turning in homework and manage to lose it between taking it out of the folder and handing it in, ask the teacher if your child may turn in all his homework by handing in the plastic folder. The teacher can remove the homework and return the folder back to your child.

314. Toss out all school papers that do not need to be saved at the end of each semester.

315. Plan assignments such as book reports and science projects on a calendar. Work backward from the due date and fill in each step of the project on the day you expect to work with your child to complete it. For example, 30th: turn in project, 29th: proofread final draft, 28th: type report. Work from the front end as well; for example, 1st: get book from library, 2nd: read pages one to twenty, 3rd: read pages twenty to forty, and so on, 15th: write outline, 17th: write introductory paragraph, 18th: write final paragraph, 19th: write paragraph two, etc.

316. Set a "get started" date for projects rather than just a deadline.

317. When plotting out project due dates on a calendar, print a blank calendar from your computer and use a pencil to write in each step on the expected day. A pencil makes it easy to erase and change if you have to revise the plan. Alternatively, you can type the calendar and reprint it each time you revise it.

318. Help your child view her project as a living thing that changes each day depending on what is accomplished and what new to-do items need to be added.

319. When your child completes a to-do on his calendar, let him cross it off. A sense of satisfaction comes from crossing things off our to-do list when we have completed them.

320. Create a grab-and-go place in your house for school items to be easily retrieved all in one location: a shelf, wall hooks, or large basket to put backpack, coat, hat, umbrella, mittens, lunch box, etc. This will save your child from having to look all over the house each morning for his necessary school items.

321. Purchase a bin or basket for each member of the family where you can toss in all the items they leave strewn about the house. You can put the basket in their room for them to put away their items. Teach your child to look in her basket if she cannot locate an item.

322. Place large colored bins or decorative baskets in your child's room to toss items into. Label bins for laundry, shoes, toys, sports items, etc., with words or photos. Once each day, usually before bedtime, your child can pick items off the floor and toss them in the proper bin. This keeps the room relatively clean and clear of clutter.

323. Dirty clothes are more likely to make it to the laundry if your child has a laundry basket in her room rather than in the laundry room or bathroom.

324. Cut down on laundry by having one basket for dirty clothes and a second basket of a different color for clothes that can be worn again. This will save you from washing clothes that your child threw in the dirty hamper because he was not motivated to put them back in the drawer or closet. Later, you or your child can put the clothes back in the drawers and closet.

325. Keep jackets, sweaters, and other bulky cold weather items off the floor by having coat hooks within easy reach for your child. ADHD children are fast-moving, impulsive, and not interested in these types of mundane tasks, so make it as easy as possible for your child to do.

326. Pick up around the house each day to keep it consistently uncluttered. Children with ADHD can learn how to keep an organized environment by following your lead.

327. Each day, help your child pick up her room and put items where they belong. This way, it can be done quickly and won't be an overwhelming task for you or your child.

328. Use a computer to quickly create a sheet of address labels to attach to your child's items that he is likely to leave behind in various places. Jackets, books, backpacks, lunch boxes, etc., are commonly lost items that can be labeled for easy return to their owner.

329. Make it easy for your child to find her clothes by labeling the outside of each drawer with a photo of the category of clothing inside. One drawer for shirts, one for pants, one for PJs, etc.

330. Keep toys in large baskets or plastic bins in your child's bedroom for an easy way to get them off the floor.

331. Keep track of important belongings by attaching a homing device to them. Press the locator button to hear the device ring so you can find it.

332. Childproof your home to prevent injuries and broken and damaged items. Children with ADHD are accident prone, so it is best to match your home decor to your child's activity level rather than his age.

333. If your child loses an important item, set up a contract detailing what she must do to earn the money to replace the lost item.

334. Make a grade log for each class for you and your child to record his grades on homework, tests, and projects. A simple computer spreadsheet with date, assignment, and grade earned will help you and your child monitor his progress in each class, rather than waiting until the end of the semester to be surprised at grades.

335. Organize your child's school records in one large three-ring binder that you can easily find and share with teachers and professionals working with your child.

Tips for
SIBLING RIVALRY

Every family with more than one child faces sibling rivalry. Families with ADHD face more than their fair share. It is difficult for the other children in the family to live with the problems their ADHD siblings tend to cause. There is no way to wipe out sibling rivalry, but here are seventeen tips to help decrease it.

336. Create an atmosphere where you encourage siblings to love and protect one another.

337. Talk repeatedly about the value of a sibling being the one person your children will have with them for their entire lives.

338. Praise all your children for any positive interaction they have with one another.

339. Recognize and thank your children for leaving the other one alone and not annoying each other.

340. Listen to each of your children's complaints about their siblings. Let them vent their frustrations without telling them "it's not that bad."

341. Do not play detective to try to find out who did what to whom. Adopt the approach of "what is the problem that needs to be solved?"

342. Involve your kids in the problem-solving process. Children will be more likely to cooperate with solutions for getting along with their siblings if they help create the remedies.

343. Establish rules for your family about getting along. Rules such as "no hitting in our family" should apply to everyone in the household.

344. Help your children learn conflict resolution by teaching them the "win-win" strategy where both parties come to an agreement they can live with, rather than one child winning and the other losing.

345. If you referee now, you will referee forever. Instead, teach your children how to verbalize their upset and work out a solution with one another.

346. Parents who are judge, jury, and executioner have children who do not get along with one another. Instead of deciding which child to punish, teach your children that any time they have a conflict that ends up in rule-breaking behavior, they will both have a consequence. This helps them learn to work things out rather than trying to get their sibling in trouble.

347. Discourage tattling. Siblings who tattle are hoping to get their sibling in trouble and put themselves in the favored position. Teach them instead to ask for your help to solve a problem rather than tattle.

348. Decrease sibling jealousy by offering an individualized token economy or behavior chart to all the children so every child gets to earn rewards and privileges.

349. Schedule special alone time with each child so they can enjoy you without the competition or annoyance of their siblings.

350. Try to enforce the rules for all the children in the family and not let the child with ADHD get away with blatant rule-breaking.

351. If your non-ADHD children do not want to participate in the token economy or behavior chart you create, make individual contracts for them to earn special rewards or privileges.

352. Encourage siblings to find the good in one another by starting a "caught ya!" reward program. Each time one child finds his sibling doing something nice or appropriate, he points it out to you. He gets a point for recognizing the good behavior, and his sibling gets a point for doing the behavior. Do not act annoyed if they do it a lot at first. Better they annoy you with praising one another than fighting with each other.

Tips for STUDYING

For most children with ADHD, studying for a test is one of the most torturous experiences they can imagine. Their symptoms prevent them from having the perseverance and motivation to study. They have little interest in memorizing information and an incredibly low tolerance for boredom. Children with ADHD have tremendous challenges starting and sticking with studying. They simply won't do it on their own and absolutely require their parent's help. Developing study skills comes at a remarkably slow pace, which means parents will have to help their children study throughout elementary and middle school. The combination of making studying fun and the promise of immediate rewards is the key to getting your child to study. These eighteen tips will get you started on putting some fun into studying.

353. Accept that your child cannot study alone and requires your help.

354. Set your mind to helping your child study instead of pushing him to do it alone.

355. Help your child study for a test by taking turns reading aloud small sections of the study material. When the reader gets to the end of the section, she quizzes the listener on the information. This way, your child is learning whether she is the reader or the listener.

356. Flash cards are the most effective study tool for almost any subject and will make studying for tests a breeze. Help your child make flash cards as she reads her textbook. Help her write one fact per index card. On the back of the card, help her write a question that pertains to that fact.

357. Once your child has made his index cards from the chapter, he will never have to look at that chapter again. When it comes time to studying for the test, he only has to use his flash cards.

358. When writing index cards for studying, it is less important who writes the card and more important that it gets written. If your child has great difficulty with writing the index cards, focus instead on him helping to select the facts and making up the questions for you to write.

359. Help your child organize her index cards so they are a useful tool for studying. Label each one with the subject and chapter. Collect the cards together by chapter, wrapping each with a rubber band, and store them in an index card box, shoebox, or even a sandwich baggie.

360. Use a different color index card for each subject to help your child stay organized.

361. Substitute flash cards for cards in board games. Use your child's flash cards to replace those of any version of Trivial Pursuit and turn studying into a fun game.

362. Incorporate study time with playtime. Play any game, and when one of you makes a wrong move or loses a turn, you have to answer a question from the flash cards. Your child is learning even when you are the one answering the question.

363. Play card games while studying. For example, when playing Go Fish, when either player has to "go fish," he not only takes a card as usual, but also must answer a question from the flash cards.

364. Take flash cards with you everywhere you go. Use them for short study bursts, such as when waiting for your food to arrive at a restaurant.

365. Let your child quiz you with the flash cards. She learns even if you are the one answering the questions.

366. Let your child move around while you quiz her with flash cards. She can swing, jump rope, bounce a ball, or jump on a trampoline while you quiz her.

367. Use any quiz-show format to make a study game out of flash cards.

368. Turn studying into a news show, with your child interviewing you using his flash cards. He can also pose as a reporter giving facts from the flash cards. Videotaping the show will not only be fun for him, but it also gives you one more fun way to help him learn the information.

369. Increase memorization of facts or definitions by having your child draw a picture of what she's studying.

370. Increase memorization of lists of items by teaching your child how to create mnemonics, such as "My Very Educated Mother Just Served Us Nachos" to remember the order of the planets: Mercury, Venus, Earth, Mars, Jupiter, Saturn, Uranus, Neptune.

Tips for
TECHNOLOGY

Technology offers wonderful opportunities that today's parents did not have the advantage of as children. Electronic devices can be used in the classroom and at home for accommodations to make tasks easier for children. Children with ADHD are especially attracted to technology, making it the ideal motivator to encourage them to cooperate, do their chores, and complete their homework. Alongside their love of technology comes the opportunity for family conflicts. Some children with ADHD behave as if they are "addicted" to TV, computers, and video games. These twenty-nine tips can help you use technology to your advantage and prevent it from being a source of conflict.

371. Use noise-reducing headphones or earplugs to screen out noise and decrease distractibility in the classroom and during homework.

372. Play a white-noise machine to block minor distracting noise during homework time.

373. Use a digital timer during homework, chores, and tasks to show your child how many minutes she has left to complete her task.

374. Make use of the cell phone by setting the alarm as a reminder for tasks.

375. Use a computer for typing in place of handwriting.

376. Use voice-recognition software for your child to dictate his report and the computer will type it for him. He can go back and edit when he is done dictating.

377. Middle school and high school students can use a laptop in place of handwritten notes.

378. Use a digital voice-memo recorder to record reminders and homework. Most cell phones have a voice-recording feature.

379. Ask your child's teacher if she would be willing to email a daily or weekly homework assignment list to parents.

380. Use a computer calendar program to organize your child's schedule of homework, projects due, and activities.

381. Color-code your child's school subjects on the computer calendar to make it easier to see what she has to do.

382. Use a vibrating watch alarm or vibrating cell phone alarm to set a timer for task reminders.

383. Allow television only as a reward. A good rule of thumb is ten points per half hour.

384. Limit the amount of TV your child watches per day, but also remember that television can be one of the most motivating rewards to gain compliance. Do not be so strict with television that your child has little motivation to comply.

385. Plan your child's television schedule ahead of time, selecting what is age-appropriate.

386. Record favorite programs and allow your child to watch them as a privilege he pays for with his tokens/points.

387. Make a weekly television schedule with your child and post it near the television so your child sees when and what she will be able to watch.

388. Give your child a five-minute warning before the television is turned off. Children with ADHD tend to be highly reactive to changes in activities that come without warning, especially TV, computer, and video games.

389. If your child refuses to turn off the TV, warn him that if he does not turn it off when you've asked him to, any time he continues to watch it now will be deducted from his TV-watching time tomorrow.

390. If your child repeatedly refuses to turn off the TV, you can take the remote control and turn it off yourself instead of arguing. Keep possession of the remote if this is a frequent occurrence.

391. Control your TV when you are not home. This means locking channels with inappropriate content.

392. Television can be a good teaching tool. Watch programs with your child that are educational, teach good moral lessons, and have positive messages.

393. Limit the amount of news your child watches on TV and hears on the radio. Children do not have the ability to put the negative content of the news into the bigger picture of the world, and they can sometimes worry that what they hear on the news will happen to them.

394. Use video game/computer game time as a reward for compliance. A general rule of thumb is ten tokens/points per half hour.

395. Do not allow unlimited gaming/computer time. ADHD children are particularly prone to behave as if "addicted" to electronic games and will play to the exclusion of other activities.

396. Allow a fixed amount of gaming/computer time per day. Psychologists have not yet agreed on what is an appropriate amount each day. Recommendations range from half an hour to no more than two hours, but this will vary from family to family. You may want to allow more time on weekends.

397. If your child refuses to close down a video/computer game, deduct tomorrow's time for as long as she refuses.

398. If your child will simply not comply with closing down a video/computer game, you have the option of putting a timer on the electrical outlet that will shut down the computer automatically.

399. If your child repeatedly sneaks gaming/computer time when you are not home, take the cord with you so he cannot turn the machine on. He can earn the cord back by cooperating with your gaming/computer rules for one week straight with a 100 percent success rate.

Tips for BEDTIME

Bedtime can present nightly challenges. All children have occasional nights when they resist going to bed, get up repeatedly, or have trouble falling asleep. These are common occurrences for children with ADHD. We do not know why insomnia is so common in children with ADHD. Current theories suggest that the brain's circadian rhythm is different in children with ADHD, making them wired to be night owls. You can't change a child's biology, but you can use these forty-six tips to create a pleasant bedtime routine and increase the chance of your child having a good night's sleep.

400. Have a set routine for bed where your child does the same tasks each night. Children who know what is expected of them at bedtime are more likely to go along with the routine.

401. Limit bedtime tasks to only those necessary for going to sleep and prepping for the next day, such as bathing, getting into jammies, brushing teeth, and picking out clothes for the next day. Do not add chores or other tasks.

402. Create a positive activity each night before bed after nighttime tasks are completed. Reading a story, cuddling and talking, watching a TV show, or playing a board game are favorite activities that motivate children to get ready for bed.

403. Have the same bedtime for each school night. A consistent bedtime will lead to consistent cooperation at night.

404. Before lights out, talk with your child about the good things he did today and praise him so he has positive feelings right before he falls asleep.

405. Keep bedtime talk positive. If you review the day's events, focus on the good. Any mention of things that went wrong can be treated lightly with, "You can try again tomorrow."

406. Avoid talking about problematic behavior at bedtime. You want your child to fall asleep with positive thoughts and feelings. However, if your child wants to talk about a problem or her misbehavior at bedtime, allow her to do so. Just keep your comments encouraging and loving so she falls asleep feeling hopeful that this behavior won't happen again.

407. Bedtime is a common time when children open up and talk about their day, their feelings, and their problems. Be sure to have your routine structured so you have time to listen.

408. Reading to your child in bed is a nice way to end the evening, even if the day has been rough.

409. Set a time limit or book limit to prevent the "Just one more story!" begging.

410. Use the reading of a story as a reward for your child getting into bed on time. Subtract any delays from his story time. If he is five minutes late in getting to bed, then story time is cut short by five minutes. Do not use this as a punishment, but just a matter-of-fact occurrence.

411. A night-light can be a sense of security, even for an adolescent.

412. Learn what helps your child fall asleep easily. A back rub, soothing music, a story, and a television with a sleep timer to shut off are common sleep inducers for some children.

413. If your child has a difficult time falling asleep, do your best not to fight with her about it. Many children with

ADHD biologically have a very difficult time falling asleep through no fault of their own.

414. Accept that you cannot "make" your child go to sleep. You can set limits that she must stay in bed, but you cannot force her to fall asleep.

415. Children who simply cannot fall asleep still need to remain in bed. Provide your child with quiet options that she can do while lying in bed, such as reading, quietly playing with a doll or stuffed animal, or listening to a book on tape.

416. Talk to your child about his ideas for staying in bed when he has trouble falling asleep. Allow reasonable ideas, such as playing with a toy, reading, or watching television for a fixed period of time.

417. Have your child lie down and read a book rather than sitting up. He may fall asleep faster this way.

418. Look to your child's medication as a potential cause of sleep problems. Insomnia is one of the most common side effects of stimulant medications. If your child's insomnia began or increased after starting or changing medications, talk to your child's prescribing physician.

419.   If your child does not adapt to medication and continues to have sleep problems, you will be faced with deciding which is more important to you: your child having better attention and concentration, or consistently getting a good night's rest.

420.   Be certain your child is getting enough sleep. Children require more sleep than adults, and children with ADHD may need more than nondisordered children. According to the National Sleep Foundation, children ages three to five require eleven to thirteen hours of sleep, five- to ten-year olds require ten to eleven hours, and ten- to seventeen-year-olds need eight and a half to nine and a half hours.

421.   Put your child to bed on time. If you are frequently putting your child to bed past the set time, you need to alter the evening routine so bedtime is consistent.

422.   Find out why your child does not want to go to bed and create a logical solution. If he is afraid of the dark, let him have a night-light or leave the hallway light on. If noises scare him, play quiet background music, or use a sound machine/white-noise machine. If he is afraid of monsters, assure him they were removed from his room before bedtime.

423.   Fridays, Saturdays, and holidays are special days and provide opportunities for your child to earn the privilege of staying up late. If she has gone to bed on time Sunday through Thursday, she can earn the reward of staying up late on Friday and Saturday. The older the child, the later she can stay up. A seven-year-old can stay up thirty to sixty minutes later; a twelve-year-old, sixty to ninety minutes later; a teenager, two to three hours later.

424. If your child has consistent difficulty sleeping, keep to a regular sleep and wake schedule seven days a week and forgo allowing a later bedtime on the weekends.

425. Remove distractions at bedtime so you can focus on your child. Turn the television off and let phone calls go to voice mail.

426. Wind down the activity level as the evening progresses. Unless you find that your child falls rapidly asleep after roughhousing or active play, keep it calm in the household the last two hours before bedtime.

427. Prevent your child from getting out of bed to ask one more question by having a pleasant chat before he falls asleep. Before you leave his room, ask him, "Is there anything else you want to talk about?"

428. Prevent your child from getting out of bed for the toilet, a drink of water, a question, etc., by anticipating all the things that cause her to get out of bed. Have her use the toilet right before she gets into bed. Next to her bed, put all the items you know she will ask for, such as water, flashlight, stuffed animal, book, clock, music, etc.

429. Prevent your child from getting out of bed to do something he forgot by making a checklist of bedtime things to do. Before your child gets into bed, go over the list with him: e.g., clothes laid out—check, backpack by door—check, lunch packed—check.

430. Prevent your child from repeatedly getting out of bed by telling her you will check on her in five minutes, and if she thinks of something she needs, she must wait until you check on her. Your child may need five-minute checks for ten, twenty, even thirty minutes. As she gets better at staying in bed, you can decrease the number of times you check on her and increase the number of minutes between checks.

431. Prevent your child from getting out of bed by using a baby monitor that your child can use to call you if he needs to. Give him a list of acceptable reasons to call you.

432. For a child who resists getting into bed, slip a surprise under her pillow that she can find only after she is in bed. The surprise should be small, such as a sticker, collector card, poker chip worth extra points, or coupon for staying up fifteen minutes later on the weekend.

433. Help your child relax once he is in bed with a physical touch he enjoys, such as light back scratching or a gentle back rub.

434. Quiet, soothing music can provide a way for your child to relax and fall asleep.

435. Teach your child to sleep in his own bed as soon as you decide he is ready. This is far easier than breaking the habit after he has been sleeping in your bed for months or years.

436. If your child finds her way into your room at night, return her to her bed with a quick kiss and rapid exit. You can be kind, but do not linger in her room; otherwise, she will quickly learn that she can get you to stay in her room at night.

437. Remove lights that might keep your child awake. Use an alarm clock with a variable light so your child can dim and lower it as needed.

438. If light distracts your child, try an eye mask to block out light.

439. If sound distracts your child, try earplugs. Even background noise can distract some children.

440. Pay attention to what your child is wearing on nights when he sleeps well and nights when he is restless. Some fabrics can be irritating to children, but they may not be able to identify why they feel bothered or are restless. Nylon and other synthetics can make children sweat and toss and turn. Flannel pajamas and sheets may be too hot for some children, even in the cold of winter.

441. Check the temperature of the bedroom for comfort. A room that is too hot or too cold may wake your child or cause restless sleep.

442. A fan set on low may help keep a room cool and provide a rhythmic humming sound that soothes your child to sleep.

443. Teens with ADHD will be more challenging at bedtime, as they will want to create their own schedule and stay up late. Work out a reasonable routine with your teen that ensures enough sleep and gives some freedom of choice.

444. *Harmonic Sleep* is a CD with subliminal harmonic music that can lull your child to sleep.

445. Hemi-Sync's *Sound Sleeper* CD sends a different signal to each ear with headphones to induce sleep.

446. Pillowsonic is a pillow with built-in speakers that plays music audible only to the person sleeping on the pillow, making it a good choice for siblings who share a room.

Tips to Help Your Child Excel in School

Tips for the CLASSROOM

The classroom can present numerous opportunities for your child to get distracted, lose focus, fidget, be impulsive, and disrupt his classmates. It is all too easy for a child with ADHD to lose self-esteem when he is frequently reprimanded by the teacher and looked upon negatively by his peers. Fortunately, the classroom is one of the easiest places to use accommodations to help your child succeed. Share these twenty-two tips with your child's teacher so you can work together to make school a place your child looks forward to going.

447. Meet with the teacher early in the school year to let her know what behavior challenges your child has so she can understand and work with your child instead of against him.

448. Do not wait until the teacher calls you with a problem to let him know your child has ADHD. It is not fair to the teacher or your child.

449. Do not think the teacher won't know your child has a disorder if you keep it secret. The teacher may not know it is ADHD, but she will surely know your child is having problems.

450. At the beginning of the school year, invite the teacher to talk with you about your child as often as she feels is necessary.

451. Provide your email address and cell phone number to make it easy for the teacher to communicate with you.

452. Keep your requests for the teacher quick and easy to implement. He will be far more likely to implement a behavior-management technique if he can do it quickly and easily and not have it interfere with the running of his classroom.

453. Work with the teacher to give a sense of control to your child if he is having frequent and serious behavior problems in the classroom. Children with severe ADHD can feel trapped in a classroom with no means to escape, which can result in highly disruptive behaviors. Allowing this type of child to leave his desk when he feels overwhelmed or out of control can prevent serious behavior problems that disturb his classmates and teacher.

454. Be realistic about your child's behavior problems. Sometimes even though ADHD children are very smart, their behavior is simply too problematic for them to remain in the mainstream classroom.

455. A special education classroom designed for children with behavior issues might be better for your child's sense of well-being, daily happiness, and academic achievement than a mainstream classroom if he is frequently in trouble.

456. For children with frequent behavior problems in the classroom, a daily behavior chart the teacher fills out can significantly improve conduct. Choose three behaviors for the chart. Select one with which she will have guaranteed success so she earns at least one point every day. Select a second behavior that is a tiny bit of a challenge for her. Select the third as the one that is most problematic. She earns one point for each successful behavior. If she succeeds on all three, then she earns three bonus points for 100 percent success. She can trade the points in for a reward and/or a privilege that day. This is most effective if the teacher, not the parent, reviews the chart with your child at the end of the day and gives the reward. You can praise your child when she shows you her chart each day, but let the teacher be in charge of the review and rewards.

457. Understand that children with ADHD interrupt and blurt out the answers because of their fear that they will forget what they want to say. Their working memory, the ability to hold a thought in their mind while they wait, is typically poor. Over the years, your child is likely to receive lower grades on her report card for classroom behavior due to repeated interrupting. Expect this to happen and don't punish your child for it.

458. Teachers can help your child work on her ability to stop interrupting and blurting out answers by sometimes calling on your child first. This will not only give your child a sense of esteem from getting to demonstrate her knowledge, but it will prevent her from disrupting the class.

459. Parents can ask their child's teacher to help ADHD children develop the ability to wait their turn by telling the class: "I will call on Andrew first, then Clarissa, and then Miguel."

460. Teachers can help ADHD children learn to hold their answers in their heads while they wait for their turn to be called on by telling the class what the question is and prompting the students to write down their answers. For example, "I am going to ask the class what the four characteristics of mammals are. I want everyone to write down their answers, and then I will ask you to raise your hand and give me one characteristic."

461. For late elementary and older children, teachers can help students with ADHD control their blurting out answers by telling them to keep a piece of paper out and jot down their answers, or a short clue to their answer so that when they are called on, they can look to their note as a reminder.

462. When students blurt out the answers, teachers can still praise them and at the same time remind and encourage them to wait their turn. For example, "That's the right answer! Good job! Next question, try to remember to wait until I call on you."

463. Remember that impulsivity is a primary symptom of ADHD and is not going away no matter how skilled the teacher is. Your child's teacher will have to work with it.

464. Ask for your child to sit up front close to the teacher to increase the amount of time he is paying attention.

465. Ask for your child to be seated next to a student who can be a positive role model for behavior and working on classroom assignments.

466. Ask for your child to be seated away from obvious distractions such as doors, windows, and talkative students.

467. Fidgety, restless children may be less distracting to their peers and classroom if they are periodically allowed to sit in the back of the class where their squirming will not distract others.

468. Homeschooling is an option for children who are not succeeding in a traditional school. Consider what advantages your child might experience if homeschooled, such as tolerance for ADHD symptoms, freedom from ridicule from peers, flexibility in assignments, and arts, music, and drama that have been removed from many schools. For more information, see www.homeschool-curriculum-and-support.com.

Tips for WORKING WITH TEACHERS

Your child's teacher is your ally. The better a relationship you can establish with your child's teacher, the better the year will go for your child, the teacher, and you. Teachers choose this profession because they love children and want to help them learn and succeed. These twenty-six tips will provide you with ways to assist the teacher with helping your child to succeed.

469. Let your child's teacher know the first week of school that your child has ADHD. It is unfair to both child and teacher to keep this hidden until the teacher figures it out on her own. After that, send a short one-page letter to the teacher and list three to five techniques that worked well for your child in last year's classroom.

470. At the beginning of the school year, provide your child's teacher with a chart of behaviors that are likely to occur in the classroom and methods that have been successful in managing them in the past. Divide your chart into three columns: one column for problems your child has, including learning, social, and behavioral; one column for ways to prevent the problems from occurring in the first place; and one column for ways to resolve the problems when they occur.

471. Provide your child's teacher with ways to communicate with you. Give her your cell phone and home phone numbers and your email address. The easier you make it for the teacher to share information with you, the more likely she will be to keep in contact more frequently.

472. Empathize with the teacher when he reports the difficulties he is having with your child. Showing you understand what he experiences with your child will go a long way in eliciting his help.

473. Avoid being defensive about your child's behavior. Teachers will go the extra mile if they see that you are working with them toward the same goal.

474. Think carefully before you hand your child's teacher information about ADHD. While any adult could benefit from learning more about the disorder, it can accidentally send a message that you presume the teacher does not know enough and that you know more. A better way would be to tell the teacher of the article or book you have found helpful and offer to loan it to her.

475. Do not demand things from your child's teacher. Few people respond positively to demands. A kind request, such as "Would you be willing to...?" works far better.

476. Keep contact with teachers short and to the point. They are very busy and won't have the time to read lengthy letters or listen to long-winded voice mails or phone calls.

477. Provide your child's teacher the necessary materials to carry out the accommodations you are requesting. This means providing her with stickers; prizes; poker chips; behavior charts; index cards with happy, neutral, or sad faces for her to circle; etc.

478. Make a partnership with the teacher; she is your ally and teammate in educating your child.

479. Keep perspective on the role of your child's teacher; he is there to teach your child academics, not be a psychiatrist, behavior therapist, or psychologist. Do not expect the teacher to solve your child's problems.

480. Volunteer at the school to establish yourself as a helper.

481. Monitor your child's 504 accommodation plan to determine if the accommodations are working or if they need to be modified.

482. Speak positively about your child's teacher so that your child respects her and cooperates with her.

483. Look for common ground between your child and her teacher. Children are often more motivated to do well in class if they like the teacher. Having something in common with her teacher can encourage your child to have positive feelings toward him.

484. Ask the teacher to privately meet with your child so they can create a secret signal the teacher can use to prompt your child to pay attention or to get his behavior back under control. This helps your child not become the center of attention for problematic behavior in the classroom. Your child will be more interested if he helps design the secret signal. The teacher may tug on her earlobe, cross her arms, write the time on the chalkboard, or various other easy to perform actions that won't let the other students know she is focusing on your child.

485. Ask your child's teacher if he would be willing, at times, to use a general prompt for the classroom instead of singling out your child, even if your child is the only one off-task or doing something inappropriate.

486. Ask for an extra set of textbooks to keep at home to eliminate the problem of your child forgetting her books, either accidentally or on purpose.

487. Ask your child's teacher if she would be willing, at times she deems it appropriate, to ignore your child's minor misbehaviors. This will help decrease the chance of your child becoming the "bad" kid in the classroom who is always in trouble.

488. Ask your child's teacher if he would be willing to use visual cues for appropriate behaviors he wishes your child to engage in, such as raising his hand if your child begins to blurt out or interrupt, a finger to the lips if your child is talking to his neighbor, and a finger to the ear if your child is not listening.

489. Ask your child's teachers for a weekly progress report to check off what homework was turned in, the grade earned, and what test scores he earned.

490. Make it easy for the teacher to complete a weekly report by designing them and printing them for her.

491. Ask your child's teacher if your child can be allowed to squirm and fidget without reprimand. Few children with ADHD can control their restless need to wiggle, and repeated prompts to sit still will quickly create a negative teacher-child interaction.

492. Ask permission for your child to have a fidget object, such as a squishy ball or a squeezable stress ball.

493. Ask your child's teacher if he would allow stretch breaks in between subjects to help give attention to the closure of one activity and the start of a new one. This can help make transitions easier for your child.

494. Thank your child's teacher for any effort she makes to help your child.

Tips for
SPECIAL EDUCATION

ADHD wreaks a lot of its havoc in the classroom. Fortunately, there are many laws to ensure children with ADHD are educated properly and get the services they need. A large percentage of children with ADHD receive special education services. If your child is having academic problems, then special education may be the answer. There is a lot to know about navigating your way around the world of special education. These fifty tips provide you with the most important pieces of information.

495. If your child is seriously struggling with school or homework, write a letter to the principal asking for a special education evaluation to determine if she qualifies for services. You will be notified of each special education meeting to discuss your child with the school.

496. Learn the laws for special education so you are an informed consumer. Wrightslaw (www.wrightslaw.com) is an informative website about special education law and advocacy.

497. Forget the rumors of special education being a place to stigmatize children. Schools have come a very long way in meeting the needs of special education students without stigmatizing them.

498. Look closely into the special education programs offered at your child's school. You may be pleasantly surprised at what they have to offer.

499. Do not assume a mainstream classroom is better than a special education classroom. Many children with ADHD perform far better in a full-time special education class with a teacher who is experienced in working with this disorder.

500. Understand that having ADHD does not mean your child automatically qualifies for special education. The disability must interfere with your child's ability to access and benefit from his education.

501. Know your child's rights for special education, but do not use that knowledge to be offensive. Instead of saying, "I know my rights!" you will receive a better response with "I know we have sixty days to get Monica tested. When do you think we can get her scheduled?"

502. Be aware that the process of qualifying for special education takes time. First, a plan has to be written that details what the assessment process will be. Once you agree, your child will then be assessed. Finally, a meeting is held to go over the results and determine if special education is appropriate, and if so, what the plan will be. This process can take several months.

503. Get acquainted with the IEP process. An IEP is an individual education plan available to children in public schools who have a disorder that is interfering with their ability to benefit from their education. This may provide a full-time special education class, resource class, one-to-one aide, or a variety of methods to assist your child.

504. Know that a 504 accommodation plan is an alternative to an IEP if your child has some challenges in the classroom and/or with homework that might be addressed with some simple accommodations and modifications. A helpful chart of accommodations can be found in *The ADD & ADHD Answer Book* by Susan Ashley.

505. Be realistic about the number of 504 accommodations you ask for. There are over one hundred helpful accommodations, which would be impossible for anyone to implement.

506. Asking for three to ten accommodations is a realistic goal that your child's teacher can likely carry out.

507. Involve your child in creating the 504 accommodations you will ask for. Ask her what she thinks would help her meet the challenges she is having.

508. Be specific when you provide information to the special education team. Instead of vague information, such as "Graham takes all night to get his homework done," provide more specific statements, such as "Graham takes two hours to write his twenty spelling words. He takes usually one hour to read only five pages in his books. He has no trouble with doing any of his math."

509. Bring to the special education meeting a written list of observations of your child's ability to do homework, complete work in class, follow school rules, behave on the playground, complete extended homework projects, write down his homework, and turn in his homework.

510. Come prepared with a list of ideas that you think might be helpful for your child, including both ideas for the classroom and for homework.

511. Create a special education notebook that includes report cards, annual academic achievement test scores, notes from teachers, IEPs, test scores and reports, 504 accommodation plans, and all other written documents related to your child's education.

512. Document all contact with the school and keep it in your special education notebook.

513. Organize your child's special education notebook by category and file documents in order by date so it is easy to read your child's history from year to year.

514. If your child will be asking for extra time on the SAT or accommodations in college, she will have to provide proof that her disorder has existed for many years. Your special education notebook should provide the necessary documentation.

515. View the special education meeting as a planning meeting to help your child, rather than a fight between you and the school.

516. Whatever your attitude is that you bring with you to the special education meeting is what you are likely to get back from the special education team. If you go in looking for a fight, you will surely find one.

517. How hard the special education team will work for your child will somewhat depend on how they feel about you. True, they have laws they must follow, but it is human nature for people to put extra effort forward for those they feel more positively toward.

518. If you are going to tape-record the special education meeting, ask permission before you turn on the tape recorder. It is not only respectful, but also may be required by law in your state.

519. Prepare a written checklist of what you want to say, what you want to know from the special education team, and what you want to resolve by the end of the meeting each time you get together. This way, you won't forget to cover what's important to you.

520. Have a team-player attitude. View yourself as a member of the special education team, each of you working together in harmony to help your child.

521. Do not view the school as an adversary. Any negative attitude from a parent can quickly turn the school into an enemy.

522. Remain optimistic that the special education team wants to help your child. Each team member chose a career in helping children, so assume they want to help yours.

523. Present yourself professionally. Dress for the special education meetings in conservative, business attire. Arrive early. Turn off your cell phone. Bring a pen and notepad, along with your special education notebook.

524. Give and expect mutual respect from the special education team.

525. Advocate but do not aggravate. You will catch more flies with honey than vinegar.

526. Special education meetings can be intimidating to parents. Expect that you will feel a bit anxious. Do your best to become knowledgeable, come prepared, and try to remain relaxed.

527. If you find yourself feeling upset or on the brink of tears or words you will later regret, ask for a change in topics

("This is a hot issue for me; can we come back to it?") or ask for a short break ("Would it be possible to take a five-minute break?").

528. Know that you do not have to sign the IEP or 504 plan. If you have any concerns or hesitations, you are within your right to state that you would like to take some time to review the plan and get back to the special education team later.

529. Ignore intimidation. Most special education meetings go smoothly, as the special education team wants to help your child, so there is little need to worry. If you feel intimidated, first consider that it might just be your own anxiety and not anything the special education team is doing to you.

530. Do not act on intimidation. If you do end up feeling intimidated, take that as a clue that you probably are not getting what you think your child needs and you are probably feeling pressure to agree to a plan you dislike. This is a good time to postpone signing the special education plan and take it home for review.

531. Do not assume a private school will be better than a public school. Many public schools have excellent programs for children with ADHD.

532. Be aware that private schools by law do not have to provide any special education services or 504 accommodations for children with ADHD. Unless a private school can cater to the needs of an ADHD child, it may not be the best educational setting.

533. If your child needs special education, give great consideration to having your child evaluated by a private psychologist. A private evaluation provides extensive testing that the school is not obligated to perform.

534. Understand that the school's evaluation will not result in a diagnosis. The evaluation is designed to only answer the question "Does this child qualify for special education?"

535. Keep realistic expectations of what the school can do for your child. Schools are there to educate children. It is up to you to do everything else, either yourself or by providing outside services to your child.

536. Accept the idea that special education programs are not sufficient to meet your child's every need. You will most likely have to find additional services outside the school setting.

537. Realize that a 504 and IEP guarantees your child equal opportunity for success. This does not mean your child is guaranteed to succeed. That is up to you and him.

538. If your school denies your child a special education evaluation or if they evaluated but denied services, your next step is to request a second meeting. Bring a special education advocate or special education attorney with you to this second meeting. The Council of Parent Attorneys and Advocates provides an online directory.

539. Approach special education meetings with the mantra, "First time alone, okay; second time alone, no way." Consider an education advocate if your child has been denied special education, or if you believe the services offered are inappropriate or inadequate. Do not continue to try to get the plan that you want on your own, as you will only be wasting your child's valuable education time.

540. If your child is denied services after the second meeting, your next step is to request a due process hearing if you believe that your child does qualify. Simply ask the special education team for the written information on due process hearings. By law, they are obligated to give you this information.

541.   A due process hearing means you need to hire a lawyer. Do not go into a legal proceeding without legal counsel. The school will have a lawyer; you should too.

542.   Do not threaten to sue the school. If you do not get the services you feel your child needs, politely say that you want to review the special education plan before signing, and you will get back to the team. Go home and contact a special education advocate or lawyer.

543.   If you will be bringing a special education advocate or lawyer to the special education meeting, inform the team of this ahead of time. The special education team will respond more positively if they feel they have not been blindsided by a surprise.

544.   Hiring a special education advocate or lawyer sets up an adversarial situation, so be do not be surprised if the special education team is more cautious with you. Continue being your polite self, and inform your advocate or lawyer if any inappropriate actions have been taken against you or your child.

Tips for EXTRACURRICULAR ACTIVITIES

Extracurricular activities are an important part of a well-balanced life. Many children with ADHD have trouble fitting in with their peers in traditional extracurricular activities. Inattentiveness may make them poor soccer and baseball players. Hyperactivity and impulsivity could annoy the other children in Scouts. Their passion for computer and video games may make it difficult to get them out of the house. These challenges simply mean you have to think a bit outside the box to find your child extracurricular activities. These twenty-eight tips can help you find activities that will suit your child.

545. Extracurricular activities are for fun. If your child is not having fun, there is no point in pushing him to try harder or stay in the activity.

546. Team sports can be too hard on some children with

ADHD. If your child does not enjoy it and seems to always be in trouble with the coach and his peers, he may not be in the right activity.

547. Fathers, in particular, may have a difficult time giving up the dream of their child being on a team and gaining the benefits that come with the experience. If your child cannot function well on a team and is chronically unhappy having to play team sports, she will not benefit from the experience, no matter how much you push.

548. Individual sports may be better for children who do not do well with team sports.

549. Consider diving, swimming, track and field, cycling, mountain biking, gymnastics, dance, martial arts, bowling, horsemanship, and golf as alternatives to team sports. These can provide just as much benefit as a team sport.

550. For children who do not enjoy or do well in sports but still want to be part of a team, consider asking the coach to create a role for them as the stats keeper, team photographer, or equipment manager.

551. Get your child outdoors to play. Recent research has verified what parents have known for centuries: playing outside is good for children's mood and behavior.

552. Provide outdoor free play so your child has time to enjoy his energy and be free of rules and structure (other than safety rules, of course).

553. Do not use removal of extracurricular activities as a punishment. The benefits derived from these far outweigh what your child will gain from losing the privilege.

554. Extracurricular activities do not have to be limited to sports. Hobbies are just as valuable, fun, and rewarding as sports.

555. Be creative in finding an extracurricular activity or hobby for your child. Painting, drawing, pottery, photography, crocheting, knitting, sewing, cake decorating, cooking, Civil War reenactment, movie-making, animation, acting, stand-up comedy, magic, hiking with the Sierra Club, skiing, snowboarding, ice skating, and chess are all examples of hobbies that children may enjoy and can find classes and clubs to enroll in.

556. Help your child investigate activities that she

thinks she might like. Read about the activity with your child, visit a site where the activity takes place, and let your child observe.

557. Let your child choose the activity that interests him, not what interests you.

558. Ask the activity leader if your child can have one trial visit before signing up.

559. Your child may enjoy an activity where you take classes together or do the activity in a club with parents and children.

560. Borrow or rent equipment required for extracurricular activities. Not only will you save money, but if your child drops out, you will be less inclined to get into a battle of insisting he continues to participate in an activity he does not enjoy.

561. If extracurricular activities require practice in between lessons, such as piano lessons, you may be setting up one more opportunity for battles between you and your child. Think about whether you are going to insist your child practice and how much time, effort, and upset you are willing to put yourself and your child through for the sake of practicing. Perhaps your child may enjoy taking singing lessons but does not enjoy the practicing in between. Unless she is driven to be a professional singer, let her just enjoy her lessons. She gets exposed to music lessons and neither of you have to fight about it.

562. Your child may enjoy practicing between lessons if you do it with him. Consider taking your own lesson and then having practice sessions at home together.

563. Your child may be more willing to practice her skill if you act as an audience for her.

564. Talk to the extracurricular leader before signing up your child. Be sure the leader knows what types of challenges your child may present and ask if the leader is willing and capable of managing them.

565. Encourage pleasure in extracurricular activities rather than success. Many children with ADHD have self-esteem so low that they cannot tolerate what they perceive as failure and they want to give up immediately. Emphasize the fun rather than the skill.

566. Extracurricular activities can be anything your child enjoys and does not have to be sports or music. Many an ADHD child has found immense happiness in a Pokemon club. Search out activities related to your child's interest. Conventions, shows, magazines, and contests provide additional opportunities for involvement.

567. Discover what your child really enjoys and find a club for it.

568. If there is no club for your child's interest, start your own. Chances are there are other children who share his interest and would be excited to be part of a club.

569. Extracurricular activities can provide a place where your child feels successful at something. This is especially important if she struggles at school and has little academic success.

570. Extracurricular activities can provide a place where your child feels he belongs socially. This is particularly important for children who are teased, bullied, and rejected at school. Activities away from school can provide an entirely different social experience.

571. Agree with your child that she will attend the extracurricular activity for a specified period of time, such as one season, earning one martial arts belt, learning one guitar song, or completing five singing lessons. Unless the activity is causing unbearable distress, make your child finish the agreed-upon contract. This will encourage perseverance and not dropping out immediately just because she is not good at something.

572. Sign up for extracurricular activities for short periods of time. A six- to eight-week duration is a good trial, rather than one year.

Tips for HOMEWORK

If only there was no such thing as homework, life would be so much happier for families living with ADHD. Some of the biggest arguments parents have with their children are over homework. It is not uncommon for children with ADHD to spend more time procrastinating, dawdling, arguing, or crying than they would spend just doing the homework. For some children, the periods of time they spend completing their homework are just about the most miserable moments of their lives. Since we can't eliminate homework, we have to learn how to work with the symptoms of ADHD. Luckily, there are many ways to make homework less stressful for you and your child. These fifty-one tips will make homework easier.

573. If your child is assigned excessive amounts of homework, ask her teacher to reduce the amount assigned. If your child's teacher is resistant to reducing homework, ask for a reduction to be written into your child's IEP or 504 Accommodation Plan.

574. Know that research on homework shows little or no increased academic achievement during elementary school and only a modest amount in middle school. It is not until high school where students are found to gain increased academic achievement from homework. These findings make it clear that homework is not a battle worth nightly arguments or the potential damage to your relationship caused by repeated conflicts with your child.

575. Be prepared to help your child with her homework. This means being available in the same room or the next room. Do not expect your child to be able to do homework alone.

576. Your child may need you to sit with him 100 percent of the time while he does his homework. If so, set your schedule to accommodate this so he gets the help he needs rather than arguing about him doing it alone.

577. Expect to help your child with her homework for several years longer than you think should be necessary (through the end of middle school is typical). ADHD children take far longer to develop the ability to work independently than non-ADHD children.

578. Put all materials necessary for homework in one well-organized container so you can put it on the table each day at homework time. This will save time looking for a stapler or eraser or pen, etc. It will also eliminate your child getting up from the table to go look for something.

579. Your child's homework container should include pencils, pens, erasers, correction fluid, Post-its, scissors, a ruler, paper clips, a stapler, staples, a staple remover, tape, colored highlighters for each subject, a calculator, colored index cards for each subject, a hole punch, plus any additional materials required by the teacher.

580. Make a backup basket with common school supplies your child is likely to need throughout the year—and likely to forget to tell you about until the night she needs them. Items might include tape, poster board, colored pens, a protractor, notebooks, book report folders, etc.

581. Homework should be done after a short snack break and before any privileges or free time.

582. Misery loves company. Your child likely does not like to do homework and will feel worse if he has to sit alone to do it. Sit with him while he works.

583. Turn off all of your child's means of outside communication during homework. This means cell phone, email, computer, and all other methods of distraction.

584. Ask your child's teacher for a second set of textbooks to keep at home to eliminate the problem of your child forgetting to bring home his books.

585. Have a few educational workbooks on hand for your child to work on when she forgets her homework. This way, she learns that she can't escape homework by forgetting to bring it home.

586. Start a homework club with at least one other parent where you swap children and help the other child with his homework. Your child will not argue with the other parent like he would argue with you.

587. Plan a fun activity for your homework club to do immediately after homework is completed so the children have something to look forward to.

588. Plan an immediate reward when homework is completed, such as playing outside, computer time, or a playdate, so your child has something fun to look forward to.

589. Offer one point for each homework problem completed. One spelling word, one point. One math problem, one point. This will increase your child's motivation to do her homework with the immediate reward of one point. She can later trade her points for rewards or privileges.

590. Use tiny food treats such as jelly beans or M&M's for immediate rewards for completing each problem or a small number of problems. If homework is done early in the afternoon, your child can eat the treats while doing his homework. If it is too close to dinnertime, he can save the treats to eat later that night for dessert.

591. Vary the location where your child does her homework. Take her to the park, the library, a lake, your backyard, a college campus, or a coffeehouse. Variety adds interest and helps beat boredom.

592. Vary where in the house your child does his homework to create some novelty.

593. Forget trying to have your child do her homework at a desk in her bedroom. She won't be able to do it alone in her room, and you will only add to her frustration, procrastination, and distractibility.

594. Have your child do his homework in a location where you are easily accessible to him, such as the kitchen counter, the dining room table, or the living room coffee table.

595. Schedule homework for a set time each day, right after school or activities. The later your child starts to do homework, the more tired she is going to be and the more difficulty she will have.

596. Set up stations around the dining room table for each subject of homework. Spelling at one chair, math at the next, science at another, and so on. Allow your child to work at a station until he feels like he wants to move, and let him rotate from station to station. This helps break up the boredom he feels, gives him a break when he is frustrated by a subject, and keeps things more stimulating by changing it up.

597. Racing the clock is a fun way to encourage your child to work faster on her homework. Place the timer so she can see it on the table and set it for a minute or two longer than the amount of time it is likely to take her to complete one task, such as twenty spelling words or ten math problems. If she finishes before the timer goes off, she earns points, a treat, or a privilege.

598. Let your child move his body while he does his homework. Sitting still in a chair is difficult for children with ADHD.

599. Allow your child to kneel on a chair or stand at the table while doing homework if she likes.

600. Use a beanbag chair for nonwriting assignments to allow your child physical comfort.

601. Try minibreaks at set intervals when your child can eat a quick snack, stretch, or use the restroom. Some children do better with minibreaks. However, other children with ADHD create more conflict by resisting returning to work. Experiment to see if minibreaks help.

602. Structure homework so that harder assignments are done first, when your child's mental energy is at its best.

603. Ask the teacher if he would be willing to send a daily email of the night's homework. This will eliminate the problem of your child forgetting to write down her homework assignment.

604. Ask the teacher to write the homework on the board

in addition to telling the class aloud. This way, your child will hear it, see it, and copy it.

605. Teach your child to write "nothing" or "no hw" to indicate that he has no homework in that subject. This way, you both will know he did not forget to write down an assignment.

606. Ask the teacher's permission for your child to use a voice-memo recorder hooked to her backpack, or on her cell phone, to record the day's homework.

607. If your child has trouble using a voice-memo recorder, ask the teacher to record it for him.

608. Ask the teacher if he can assign a row captain to collect the homework to ensure that your child does not forget to turn it in.

609. Ask the teacher to place a bin on her desk for turning in homework.

610. Ask the teacher to cut your child's amount of homework in half but still give full credit for completion. This can be written into your child's IEP or 504 plan.

611. Set a finite amount of time for your child to do homework. When the timer goes off, your child is done doing homework even if it is not complete. There is no need to spend each weeknight arguing about homework for hours.

612. Keep a log of how long it takes your child to complete each assignment so you can track which subjects are easier and which ones cause him the most difficulty. Use this information to help organize how the homework is to be done, such as most difficult first, or break it up with some easy assignments mixed in with short periods of difficult ones.

613. Share the homework time log with your child's teacher to develop a reasonable amount of homework to be assigned.

614. Use your homework time log to restructure how your child does her homework. It can help you determine which assignments to do first, which subjects need a tutor, which types of projects need additional time, etc.

615. Create a daily homework assignment sheet for your child on your computer. Make a column for each subject, the assignment, the materials needed, when it is due, when it is turned in, and the grade earned. Your child's notebook should have one for each school day.

616. Color-code your child's subjects, each subject having its own color. The color-coding provides an easy visual cue to gather all the necessary materials for each subject. Cover textbooks in the assigned color, use the color on your customized daily homework assignment sheet, use matching colored index cards for flash cards, etc.

617. Hire a tutor. This will be the best money you've ever spent. A high school or college student is often all your child needs. The tutor should be someone your child likes and wants to please and someone who is good at motivating and keeping your child on track with getting the homework done.

618. Hire a special education tutor only if your child has a learning disability. Otherwise, you are overpaying if your child simply needs someone to sit with her and keep her on task and help her organize her work.

619. If you can't hire a tutor, find another parent, swap kids, and be the tutor for the other child while the other parent tutors your child. It is free this way, and both parents save a lot of frustration.

620. Make instructions clear by writing them in large print for your child to refer to while doing an assignment.

621. Decrease careless errors by highlighting instructions for your child to refer to.

622. Use a block-out reader, a colored strip of see-through plastic that allows your child to see only the line that he is reading while the lines above and below are blocked out.

623. Photocopy one chapter at a time to read from and put the textbook aside. Having a small stack of papers is less overwhelming than an entire book. Your child will also be able to highlight and write notes on the page as she reads.

Tips for MATH

There are no real patterns in math when it comes to children with ADHD. Some love it; some hate it. For some, it comes easy, while for others, it's a struggle. The repetition required to learn math can cause resistance even for children who like the subject. Here are nine tips to make math more fun.

624. Use tangible items during math homework. Pennies, dried beans, peanuts, etc., provide a visual cue, making it easier to do the calculation, all while bringing math into the real world.

625. Use tiny treats as tangibles for your child to do her math problem. After she is done with her math, she can eat the treats. Jelly beans, M&M's, Skittles, sunflower seeds, raisins, etc., are small treats that won't disrupt her appetite. If it is too close to dinner, save the edible treats for dessert.

626.   Bring math into your child's world by making it about something he loves. Instead of asking him to multiply 8 x 3, let him solve the problem of 8 families, each with 3 brontosaurs, who are looking for a pterodactyl; how many brontosaurs will the pterodactyl have to fight off?

627.   Watch for careless mistakes such as adding instead of subtracting or putting a number in the wrong column. These are common occurrences for children with ADHD who rush through their work and do not take the time to check for errors.

628.   Prevent careless mistakes by highlighting all the addition signs in one color and all the subtraction signs in another. As your child gets older, he can do the highlighting.

629.   Teach your child to circle the math symbol before starting the problem as a visual cue and reminder that he is supposed to multiply or divide, etc.

630.   Use computer math programs to make math fun. Almost anything can be made fun if it is done on a computer.

631.   Use graph paper to keep numbers lined up and placed in the proper column.

632. Help prevent math errors with the use of a talking calculator that speaks the number and symbol pushed. The auditory feedback can be a helpful tool in decreasing errors.

Tips for READING

Reading can be a great source of pleasure for some children. Yet for many children with ADHD, it is a source of dreaded work. Even for children with high reading ability, it takes extra effort and mental energy to read, something most children with ADHD resist. Reading well is perhaps the most important academic skill your child needs now and throughout life. Almost everything we do in life requires reading, so it is an area where parents cannot drop expectations. Use these thirty-three tips to help your child learn to read and enjoy it.

633. Be sure to look at your child's annual academic achievement test scores for reading to see if it falls below average. Scores below 25th percentile warrant an evaluation for a reading disorder.

634. Children who have a lot of negative emotion about reading might have a reading disorder and should be evaluated.

635. Be sure your child has been thoroughly tested for reading disorders if she struggles. Reading ability is broken up into fluency and comprehension. Fluency tells how rapidly your child can say the words she is reading, but says nothing about whether she understands them. Comprehension tells how well your child understands what she is reading. Your child can have high fluency but low comprehension.

636. Take turns reading aloud with your child. You read one page, he reads the next.

637. Stimulate interest in the book by looking first at the cover and the title and talking about what the book is about.

638. To increase interest and comprehension, at the end of each chapter, talk with your child about what has happened in the story so far and what she thinks might happen in the next chapter.

639. Let your child read what interests him. Do not worry so much about *what* he reads but *that* he reads.

640. Let your child read the sports page in the newspaper if he loves professional sports. Reading is reading.

641. Encourage pleasure reading by subscribing to magazines about your child's interests and hobbies.

642. Allow comic, anime, and cartoon books, which may hold your child's interest more than fiction and nonfiction books.

643. Buy children's magazines, which have short stories and photographs, making reading less overwhelming than facing an entire book.

644. Photocopy one chapter at a time for your child to read. It is easier for your child to think about reading this small packet of papers rather than the entire book.

645. Photocopying chapters will allow your child to use a highlighter to mark the important points.

646. Give a tiny treat or a point at the end of each reading section. Tiny means one small piece of a small candy, one M&M, one bite of a cookie, one piece of candy corn, etc.

647. While reading textbooks, ease the transition into reading a chapter by first reading the title, all section titles, captions under photographs, graphs, charts, etc.

648. Allow your child to read aloud even if she is reading alone. Reading aloud lets her see it, say it, and hear it, giving her three modalities to learn the information.

649. Help your child learn to quietly mouth the words so that he learns to use the reading aloud technique in places where he cannot read aloud, such as the library, classroom, and during tests.

650. Allow your child to use her finger to hold her place while reading, regardless of how old she is. Many students with ADHD easily lose their place while reading.

651. Allow your child to use a bookmark to hold his place while reading to prevent his eyes from wandering.

652. Use a magnifying stick that magnifies and underlines one sentence to help your child keep her place. These can be found at knitting and craft stores.

653. Use a reading window to block out all but one or two lines on the page. These can be made by cutting out a window in a file folder.

654. Focus on one section at a time rather than an entire chapter. Put a paper clip or a sticky note at the end of a short section so your child sees he only has to read to the note or clip.

655. After each section in a textbook, talk about what the child just read to help increase comprehension.

656. Encourage your child to take notes on index cards as she reads. This not only helps with learning and memorizing the material, but can also be used to study for tests.

657. For book reports, encourage your child to take notes on index cards about the characters and events in the story as he reads. This will give him all the information he needs when it is time to write the book report. Be sure to have your child number the index cards as an easy method to keep the information in proper order.

658. If your child highly resists reading a book that her teacher selected for a book report, ask permission for your child to read a book of her choice as an accommodation.

659. Watch the movie version of a book with your child before he reads it. This will increase his ability to understand what he reads, as well as likely make the book more interesting to him.

660.   Use the reward of watching the movie version of the book after your child has finished reading the book. Many popular children's books have been made into movies, giving you an easy way to motivate pleasure reading.

661.   Increase awareness of stories by talking about how the movie and the book were different.

662.   Use books on CD to play as your child reads along. Be sure to use the unabridged version so the CD and the book are exactly the same. This allows your child to see and hear the words, making it easier for her to understand the story.

663.   Learning Ally offers more than 70,000 downloaded books. Unlimited books can be downloaded for $99 per year.

664.   National Library Service offers free loans of almost any book on cassette, or your local library may have the book you need on tape/CD.

665.   Play board games with written questions. This way, your child practices reading without knowing he is practicing reading.

Tips for SPELLING

Weekly spelling words are part of every child's education. Writing words over and over challenges the ability of children with ADHD to tolerate repetitive, boring tasks. Spelling is a vital skill and one where parents cannot be lenient. Try these eighteen tips to make spelling more fun for your child.

666. Use a Scrabble board to practice weekly spelling words.

667. Use alphabet macaroni noodles or alphabet cereal as a fun way to practice weekly spelling words. Let your child eat the cereal as a treat when he is done.

668. Use an Aquadoodle, a water-filled mat that your child can write on and erase, to practice weekly spelling words.

669. Allow your child to practice her weekly spelling words outside using sidewalk chalk.

670. Set up finger or brush painting to excite your child about practicing spelling words.

671. Buy colorful, glittery pens and markers that will make your child eager to write his spelling words.

672. Have bright, colorful paper on which your child can write her spelling words.

673. If your child puts up much resistance to writing his words on paper, but is willing to use one of the fun methods previously described to write them, ask permission from his teacher to allow him to turn in a digital photo of his spelling words written with macaroni, sidewalk chalk, or another fun technique.

674. Let your child stand, kneel, or sit on a beanbag chair while he writes his spelling words. Whatever is comfortable for him.

675. Try letting your child jump rope as she spells the words out loud to you. Rhythmic movement has been found to help children with memorization.

676. Give your child a ball to bounce as he recites the spelling words to you. The rhythm of the bouncing can help with memorization.

677. Let your hyperactive child move around while she spells out loud to you. Large motor movements such as climbing, swinging, jumping jacks, and hopscotch allow your child to move while simultaneously practicing spelling.

678. Set up a spelling course around the house or backyard where your child has to run from station to station and write or recite the spelling of one word per station.

679. Use a timer for spelling words to encourage your child to write his spelling words quickly. He can earn points or a tiny prize if he beats the clock.

680. Allow typing of spelling words if your child has fine motor problems that cause her great difficulty in writing. Be sure to turn off auto-correction.

681. Use voice-recognition software for your child to practice his spelling words. You say the word aloud to him, he spells it into the microphone, and the computer types it for him.

682. Dictionary.com is a fast and easy method for your child to become accustomed to using a dictionary to check her spelling.

683. Use rhythmic hand-clapping games while practicing spelling words.

Tips for WRITING

Writing can be a daunting task for children with ADHD for a variety of reasons. It can be difficult to simply hold the pencil or pen properly and near impossible to control the impulse to race through the assignment. Thinking of what they want to write down and holding it in their working memory long enough to get it on paper can be too difficult for many children with ADHD, who tend to quickly forget what they wanted to write. Organizing the words, sentences, and paragraphs in proper sequence can be too big of a hurdle. Writing tasks can result in procrastination and conflict between parent and child, or teacher and student. What appears as defiance may truly be caused by difficulties with writing that your child may not be able to describe to you. Use these tips to help ease the stress of writing for your child.

684.   Be aware that many children with ADHD are visual thinkers rather than verbal thinkers.

685. Tap into your child's visual abilities and have him "see" his book report like a movie. Ask him what he sees as the beginning, middle, and end of the movie, and you will then have the outline for the report.

686. For children who like to draw, sketching out ideas for a book report or essay can serve as the outline.

687. Have your child write each idea for the report on a separate index card. She can then put the index cards in order and write the report in the same order as the index cards.

688. For children who put irrelevant information in a report, have them use the movie technique and ask them if each scene fits in this movie or if it would be better in another movie.

689. Five-paragraph essays can be started by having your child trace her hand on a piece of paper and write the main idea on the pinkie finger, the summary idea on the thumb, and one idea each for the remaining three fingers. The essay can then be written from this outline.

690. Your child can dictate his essay to you and you can write it down.

691. Ask the teacher if your child may type her report on the computer instead of handwriting it.

692. Use voice-recognition software for your child to talk into a microphone while the computer types it on the screen. Your child can easily speak his thoughts and not have to worry about the challenges of actually writing with pen and paper. He can go back afterward to edit.

693. Use AlphaSmart's NEO 2 laptop to type instead of paper and pen.

694. Ask the teacher if your child can video tape her report instead of writing it. She may be excited by giving the report like a news reporter.

Tips for GRADES

Grades can be a source of conflict between parents and children with ADHD. Parents want their children to do their very best and earn the highest grades they are capable of earning; children with ADHD want to rush through their work and get the boring assignments done as quickly as possible. There are ways for parents and children to meet somewhere in the middle. These twenty-one tips can put grades in their proper perspective and take the pressure off you and your child.

695. Decrease your worry about your child's grades. Remember that 85 percent of the population is in the average range. Statistically speaking, most children are going to be B and C students.

696. Do not pressure your child to be an A student, especially if he is not A-student material. You will only frustrate him and cause a rift in your relationship.

697. Grades are not the be-all and end-all in life. Very few people have their lives shaped for them by the grades they earned in school, especially elementary and middle school.

698. Help your child monitor her progress with a weekly report card from her teacher. This will prevent a surprise report card filled with Ds and Fs at the end of the semester.

699. Get around your child forgetting to bring home weekly report cards by asking the teacher to email them to you.

700. Help your child keep track of homework turned in with a weekly homework report from his teacher.

701. Store all your child's report cards in her records notebook. They will be of great help to professionals evaluating her.

702. Increase the chance that the teacher will be willing to fill out weekly report cards and homework reports by making it easy for her. Design and print them out for her.

703. Use weekly report cards as a motivator for rewards and privileges. Assign a point value to each letter grade. For example, the plan sets an A worth thirty points, a B worth twenty, a C worth ten, a D worth one, and an F worth zero.

704. Teach your child that the brain is like the muscles in her body: the more it is worked, the more it grows.

705. Respond to your child's low grades with the philosophy that mistakes are good teachers. Your child won't be so hard on himself if you show him how he can learn from his mistakes.

706. Praise your child's efforts, not her intelligence. "You really worked hard on that project!" rather than "You are so smart!" teaches her that it is effort that counts.

707. Look for effort and attitude more than high academic grades. Right from the start in kindergarten, praise your child's effort and success and instill in him a feeling of pride in himself. Of course you are proud too, but eventually he will lose interest in earning good grades just to please you. Set the stage early so that he is working to make himself proud. "You must be so proud of yourself!" instills self-pride more than "I am so proud of you."

708. Remember, school is about the learning, not the earning (of grades).

709. Know that report cards tell you how well your child performed on the assignments, not how much she learned. Your child can earn a D in history but still know more about the subject than any of her peers.

710. Take inventory of how well your child is learning by looking at his annual academic achievement test scores. These tests measure if your child learned what he was supposed to learn during the school year. If his scores are in the average to above-average percentile, then you know he is learning even if his grades are poor.

711. Do not get emotionally attached to your child's grade. Your child's grades do not reflect your parenting ability.

712. Drop "we" from your vocabulary when you talk about your child's grades. "We" earned an A or "we" have a book report due says you are far too invested in your child's grades.

713. Worry less about your child's grades, provided she is passing, and more about her emotional and social development.

714. Remind yourself that emotional intelligence and the ability to get along with others have a far greater predictive value of success than academic grades.

715. Ask successful adults you know if they were good students. You'll likely find many who were not good students but still managed to grow up to be successful adults.

Tips for Healthy Social Interactions

Tips for
SOCIAL SKILLS

Making and keeping friends can be a challenge for children with ADHD. Their excessive activity, talkativeness, and impulsivity can make them undesirable playmates. Reading social cues and knowing how to get along with others does not come naturally to many children with ADHD. Teasing, bullying, and rejection can be constant companions for some children with ADHD. Troublemaking friends at school can result in a child with ADHD being too fearful to invite peers over, preferring solitude over risking rejection. Parents have to take a very active role in organizing social activities that foster their children's opportunities to develop lasting friendships. Not only do parents have to orchestrate their children's social lives, but they also have to teach their children specific ways to be a friend. These twenty-five tips provide ways to incorporate friendship skills into daily life.

716. Know that ADHD children are typically two to three years behind socially and thus will require supervision on playdates for several years longer than you would expect.

717. Encourage your child to invite peers for playdates or social get-togethers.

718. Plan a fun activity and ask your child if he would like to invite someone to join him.

719. If your child resists inviting anyone over to play, consider arranging the playdate yourself with the other parent. Your child may be too afraid of rejection to risk inviting someone over.

720. If your child has trouble making friends his own age, a child a few years older can be more patient and tolerant with your child and therefore a better playmate.

721. Organize a group activity for parents and children. You will be sure your child has at least one friend to come over and you will have other parents for extra supervision.

722. Keep playdates time limited so they are successful and the two children will not tire of one another and find themselves in conflict.

723. Keep playdates limited to one-on-one until your child is able to handle more than one playmate at a time. Adding a third child can be too stimulating and increases the chance of inappropriate behavior and conflicts.

724. When arranging playdates, choose activities that are fun and do not require constant interaction between the children. A structured activity will be easier for your child to manage than a simple playdate where he is left to just play. A movie, a trip to the park, rollerblading, and bike riding are activities that do not require intense interaction, but allow your child to have fun with a friend.

725. Children with ADHD often overreact when things don't go their way. Their intense emotions can unintentionally end a friendship. Remind your child that she and her friend should come ask for your help if they have a conflict they cannot solve.

726. Remind your child before the playdate that if he has a meltdown in front of his friend, that friend may not want to come over again. Encourage him to come ask for help before he has a problem.

727. Determine how much direct supervision your child needs based on her ability to get along with her playdate rather than her age.

728. Supervise your child on a playdate to help him with social skills such as sharing, taking turns, and offering his friend the choice of what to play.

729. Allow your child to play with younger children if she likes to. Younger children will look up to her, and this will help her feel good about herself.

730. Many ADHD children need help entertaining their playdates and being good hosts. Plan activities ahead of time for your child and his playdate to do.

731. Talk positively to your child when teaching her social skills. Do not point out that she has trouble with friends; she probably already knows that. Instead, keep it positive: "I am going to teach you something that will help make you a better friend than you already are!"

732. Do not try to "fix" all your child's social deficits at once. Focus on one or two social skills at a time. This will allow your child to learn a skill and try it out repeatedly.

733. Avoid using negative words to describe your child to others. Descriptors such as "liar," "manipulative," and "lazy" are critical, hurtful, and undermine your child's opportunity to feel good about himself each time he hears them.

734.   Describe your child's behaviors rather than assigning her labels. A "lazy" child is actually a child who has trouble getting tasks done. A "liar" is a child who is motivated to avoid getting into trouble.

735.   Praise your child's efforts at socialization regardless of her success level.

736.   More extracurricular activities mean more opportunities for positive social interactions.

737.   Teach your child how to introduce himself and have him rehearse it over and over at various points in time. The more comfortable he becomes with this skill, the more he increases his chances of making friends.

738.   Send your child to a summer camp specializing in ADHD. Trained camp counselors will make sure your child is included socially, practices appropriate social skills, and learns how to work out social conflicts.

739.   Provide your child with books about friendship.

740. Watch movies and TV shows with your child and talk about the friendship skills observed on screen.

Tips for
PERSONAL SPACE

Keeping inside their own physical boundaries is difficult for children with ADHD. They can get too close, touch others too much, and intrude into other people's personal space. Most children do not mean to violate others' personal boundaries; they simply are not aware of the invisible lines that most people are accustomed to not crossing. Their gross motor movements are oftentimes awkward and out of their control, so they bump into others, knock things over, and frequently trip and fall into objects or people. It is easy for others to find this annoying. Controlling their bodies and understanding where they are in physical space comes slowly for some ADHD children. Try these nine tips to help your child control where he puts his body.

741. Give your child something to hold in his hands to help prevent him from touching others. A toy, stuffed animal, pencil, squishy ball, pillow, or book will keep hands busy and out of contact with others.

742. Space out chairs so your child cannot reach the person next to her.

743. Give your child a task to do with his hands during times he is most likely to touch others. Have him draw a picture, make a list of what he wants to do over school vacation, turn the pages during story time, collect the ribbons from gifts at the party, keep a tally of the number of times people say the word "and." Almost any activity you can think of will provide a distraction from breaking physical boundaries.

744. Use cushions when sitting on the floor to help your child keep to her own personal space.

745. At school, colored masking tape can be put on the floor to outline where each child is to sit during circle time.

746. Colored masking tape can be put on the floor where each child is to stand during lineup at the beginning of the school day.

747. Teach your child that he has an invisible bubble around him that extends as far as his arms reach, and he should make sure his invisible bubble does not touch anyone.

748. Direct your child to put her hands in her pocket during times she is touching others.

749. Seek occupational therapy if your child is having significant and frequent problems with personal space.

Tips for PUBLIC BEHAVIOR

Every parent's nightmare is having their child act out in public. It is normal to feel embarrassed when your child misbehaves or has a tantrum. While most people are used to seeing toddlers have meltdowns, they are not accustomed to seeing an older child act like a toddler. Children with ADHD can be very emotionally immature and act years younger than their biological age, especially when they do not get their way. They are also very aware of how far to push at home versus in public. It takes only a few times of getting his way before your child figures out that you can't control him outside the home. It is never too late to take back control in public. These nineteen tips will get you back in charge.

750. Remind yourself that the only reason strangers are watching you and your child is to see who wins, you or the child. You get to determine the winner.

751. Take comfort in knowing that strangers watching a

showdown between you and your child are always quietly cheering for you.

752. Do not give in to your child to avoid embarrassment. Be firm and stick to your rules. Let your child know by your refusal to give in that she cannot attempt to get her way by making a public scene.

753. Ignore bystanders who might be watching you deal with your child. It does not matter what others think about your parenting. They do not know your child, so they have no basis to form valid opinions about you.

754. Make a list of problems you have encountered with your child in public, and design a way to try to prevent each problem from taking place. For example, if your child screams for a toy in the grocery store, bring a special one she can play with only on grocery trips.

755. If prevention fails, then plan a way to solve the problem ahead of time. When it happens again, you will know exactly what you are going to do.

756. Make rule cards for each place you know your child has trouble in. Read it with your child before you arrive.

757. Before you go anywhere with your child, ask her to tell you what the rules for that setting are.

758. Remind your child before you enter a public place what the consequences are of his behavior. For example: "If you do not ask me to buy you something while we are in the grocery store, you will get a piece of gum when we get back in the car. If you ask me one time to buy you something, then you do not get any gum."

759. Ask your child to repeat to you what she is expected to do, what will happen if she complies, and what will happen if she does not comply.

760. As soon as you begin to notice problem behavior, address it immediately. Ignoring it increases the chances that things will get out of control.

761. When your child begins to behave inappropriately, ask him right away what he is upset about and what he needs to solve it.

762. Do not assume you know why your child is misbehaving. Ask her why.

763. Validate your child's upset so he does not have to escalate in his behavior to make you acknowledge his feelings. "I know you are angry with me because I won't let you sit by yourself in the movie. I understand."

764. Be prepared to leave any situation if your child is behaving in an unacceptable way and nothing seems to be helping bring her back under control.

765. If your child's behavior is interfering with others around you, remove him from the situation. You will be more confident in your parenting if you do not have strangers' eyes upon you, and your child will learn that misbehaving in public means he has to leave the situation.

766. Be prepared to go home or sit in the car until the others in your group are done with the activity if your child cannot bring herself back under control. While this is frustrating and means one parent has to miss the activity, doing so only a few times will quickly make the point that misbehavior will not be tolerated.

767. If activities have to be terminated because your child cannot behave, take the other children out at a later time for a "rain check" so they can redo the activity without their misbehaving sibling. This is fair to the other children and helps teach the misbehaving child that if he cannot control himself, he will miss out on the fun and his behavior will not deprive his siblings of their fun.

768. Plan dress rehearsals for situations when you know your child will have difficulties. If he has a screaming fit every time you go to the grocery store, plan several trips to the grocery store when you do not absolutely need to shop. Do not tell your child, of course, that you are only doing a dress rehearsal. If he throws a tantrum, you can leave without interfering with your need for groceries. Go to a restaurant when you do not need a meal. Shop at the mall when you have nothing you need to buy. If your child is doing well, continue with the task and complete it, buy some groceries, eat a meal, or shop at the mall and praise him for doing a good job. Dress rehearsals prevent you from being in a situation where you let your child get away with inappropriate behavior because you have to get a certain task done. The more you have dress rehearsals, the faster you will train your child to behave in public.

Tips for SELF-ESTEEM

How a child perceives and values himself defines self-esteem. Children with ADHD can have low self-esteem due to the continual feedback from teachers, parents, and peers that they seem to almost always be doing something inappropriate. Self-esteem determines how hard we are willing to try at something, how much we are willing to risk failure, how we feel about where we fit in socially, how successful we strive to be, and how happy we are. It is a vital aspect of every child's psychology and needs to be fostered with extra effort for children with ADHD. These twenty-five tips will give you food for thought about increasing your child's self-esteem.

769. Purposely look for the good in your child and praise it.

770. Encourage your child's natural talents.

771. Focus on what is going right each day.

772. Focus on character more than behavior. A charitable and kind child is more desirable than a greedy, mean child who gets all his homework done.

773. Create opportunities for your child to engage in things in which she excels.

774. Balance difficult tasks with fun, easy activities.

775. Be sure to say "I love you" every day. ADHD children need to know that their behavior problems do not lead to them being unloved.

776. Being reprimanded multiple times each day wears down a child's self-esteem. You can help counter this by expressing your appreciation for anything positive you catch your child doing.

777. Involve your child in charity work. Helping others makes everyone feel good. Your child can donate his toys to charity, run or walk a Kiddie 1K for a charitable cause, or send 5 percent of his birthday and holiday money to a charity.

778. Be your child's "go to" person, the one person she

knows will always be there to listen to her and provide empathy, support, encouragement, and understanding.

779. Make it easy for your child to come to you with a problem or a confession about his behavior. This means being a good listener and giving him understanding and empathy, not a lecture.

780. Give unconditional love. Everyone needs one person who loves them no matter what. Be the person your child knows will love her unconditionally.

781. Open your ears and close your mouth when your child is talking to you about a problem or how she feels. A good listener is much better than a good talker when it comes to getting children and teens to open up.

782. Do not be so quick to share your experience, advice, and wisdom. Often your child just needs to express himself without having to listen to what you think.

783. We learn best by evaluating our choices and thinking about them, rather than by being told by others what they think. Instead of giving advice, ask your child what she thinks about what she did, how she feels about her choice, whether

her choice is consistent with her values, and whether she would have made a different choice if she could do it again.

784. Create a wall of fame in your house where you display your child's photos, ribbons, certificates, and awards. His bedroom is an ideal spot so he sees his success every time he goes to his room.

785. Make a scrapbook of your child's accomplishments. Items removed from the wall of fame can be permanently stored in her scrapbook. Children love to look at a book all about themselves.

786. If your child has not earned any awards, certificates, or ribbons, seek out opportunities for him to do so. Junior Ranger programs in national parks, zoos, and the Scouts provide certificates for participation, and charity walks and runs give every finisher a medal.

787. Helping your child succeed in daily tasks and rewarding her for it will build self-esteem and avoid a chronic sense of failure.

788. Know that low self-esteem places children at risk for more serious issues in their teen years. Low self-esteem can lead to depression, school failure, truancy, antisocial peer groups, smoking, alcohol use, drug use, promiscuity, and delinquency.

789. Monitor what you say to your child so you avoid highly critical, cruel, and demoralizing words you can never take back. In times of high frustration, not talking may be the best option.

790. Focus on one or two behaviors at a time. If your child is beat down by you pointing out every misbehavior and fault, he won't have enough self-esteem to try to improve.

791. Leave surprise notes with something you love about your child: "I love the way you tell jokes! Can't wait to hear one tonight when you get home."

792. Leave surprise thank-you notes for your child for ordinary behaviors she has done: "Thank you for putting your baseball equipment away yesterday."

793. Do not let your child use ADHD as an excuse for behavior. This will contribute to an identity of himself as flawed and not in control of himself. "It's true, honey, that you have ADHD, but that does not mean you cannot make good choices."

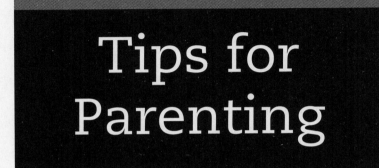

Tips for Parenting

Tips for COOPERATION

Getting an ADHD child to cooperate can seem like an endless, uphill battle that you can never win. Oftentimes, the child with ADHD is not purposely misbehaving or being noncompliant; it is just that his symptoms of ADHD make it incredibly difficult for him to do what is expected of him. He does not hear what you told him to do. Or, if he heard, he forgets. He does not remember rules and routines from day to day. He does not learn from punishment. He wants all the fun without doing the work. Adding to his difficulty cooperating is the fact that at least 50 percent of children with ADHD also have Oppositional Defiant Disorder, which dramatically increases their lack of cooperation and defiance. Getting your child to cooperate will be a daily job that won't end, but it can be made easier if you use these forty-eight tips.

794. Set your focus on "What is she doing right?" and you will find that no matter how much she misbehaves, she is cooperating far more often than not.

795.   Rejoice in the many little things your child does right. It will make the noncompliance easier to handle.

796.   Make a list of all the things your child does right. Refer to it often, especially in times of frustration to remind yourself of all the many things he does right.

797.   The more you praise and thank your child for doing the right thing, the more often he will do the right thing.

798.   Keep your praise 100% positive and do not follow praise with a negative. "I like how you cleaned your room today. See it wasn't so bad! Why can't you do that everyday?" This is a compliment followed by an insult. Stop talking about why you liked what he did and let your child enjoy the praise.

799.   One day each month, try avoiding all negative comments, ignoring all but the dangerous behaviors, and focus on praising only the good. You may be surprised by how good you feel about your child at the end of the day and pleased about how much of his behavior you can actually just let go and ignore.

800.   If your child's behavior is so problematic that it is difficult to find opportunities to praise him, put ten poker chips in your pocket in the morning as a reminder to catch him doing something right at least ten times each day. You may have to look hard and praise the most basic of behaviors, such as simply getting out of bed, sitting at the table, sitting in the car, etc.

801. Use a variety of ways to say "Thank you." "I like it when you…" "It is so helpful when you…" "I really appreciate that you…"

802. Use directives as your primary tool for telling your child what you expect her to do. A directive is a simple command that says "Do this." It is not a question, request, or invitation for negotiation.

803. Be sure your child is listening to you when you are giving a directive. If he is distracted, he will not hear you or remember what you told him to do.

804. If your child repeatedly does not follow your directives or seems to forget what you said, ask her to repeat to you what you just told her to do. This will ensure that she did indeed hear you and gives her the opportunity to put it into her memory by saying it aloud.

805. Give one directive at a time. Children with ADHD have trouble with working memory, which means they cannot hold multiple things in their minds, so even if he did listen to you, he immediately forgets what you just told him. Think of it as being similar to when you are introduced to somebody and you forget their name almost instantly. What looks like noncompliance may simply be a failure to remember what he just heard.

806. Give one directive and praise when it is completed. Then give your second directive and praise, and so on.

807. Tell your child what to do, instead of what not to do. Saying "Do not put your feet on the table" does not tell her where to put her feet. Do not be surprised when she puts her feet on the couch instead of the floor if you did not say "Please put your feet on the floor."

808. Do not punish forgetfulness. ADHD children cannot hold rules, routines, and tasks in their minds. They forget everyday rules and tasks, even though they have been doing them for months or years. Every day is a new day in their minds, and they do not know what to do unless you tell them.

809. Try your best to remain calm when your child is not cooperating. If you remain calm, your child will be more likely to remain calm.

810. Avoid using negative labels about your child's behavior. Critical words can become etched in your child's mind, and he will come to identify those pejorative words with who he is.

811. Focus on the here and now, forget yesterday's behavior, and don't predict tomorrow's. Every day with ADHD is different from the next.

812. Nothing happens until your child cooperates. If you give a directive that must be completed, then nothing else takes place until your child cooperates. If your child was told to clean his room, then he cannot do anything else until his room is clean.

813. Act as if you do not care. Oppositional defiant children may enjoy watching their parents become angry in reaction to noncompliance. If this is your child, give your directive and act as if it does not matter to you whether she complies. The more invested you are in your child cooperating, the more she may dig in her heels and refuse to cooperate as a means of retaliating, expressing her anger, and gaining control over you. If your child sees that her noncompliance has no impact on you, she is less likely to be oppositional.

814. Maintain control by giving it away to your child. "It's your choice" will be one of your most frequent phrases. When your child tells you he won't feed the dog, you respond with the consequence he will face and tell him it is his choice to cooperate or deal with the consequence. "If you do not feed the dog, that's fine: I will feed the dog and you will lose your television privileges for tonight. It's your choice."

815. Eliminate power struggles. Many acts of defiance are simply your child's urge to gain power over you. If you join her in the fight, you lose. Do not get into a battle you cannot win. Instead, use the "it's your choice" method.

816. Accept that there are some things you absolutely cannot make your child do. You cannot make your child eat, go to sleep, or quit crying. Do not insist on things you cannot enforce.

817. Always follow through with the consequence you promised when you gave your child the choice of complying or choosing the consequence. Failure to follow through destroys your power and authority.

818. Refer to your rule notebook anytime your child argues about a rule. Together, you and your child will create the rules, write them, and sign that you know what the rules are. When your child argues that he did not know he was supposed to take the trash out or face losing his computer privilege for the night, you can turn to your rule notebook.

819. Decrease the number of directives you give. Ask yourself first if the directive you are about to give is necessary. Give only those you find necessary. Giving too many directives increases the chance of opposition and defiance.

820. Help your child understand why she has to do the things you direct her to do. Ask "Why do I…?" "What would happen if…" questions, like "Why do I have you put your clothes in the hamper?" or "What would happen if I let you eat anything you wanted?" The more your child understands why she has to do things she does not like to do, the less opposition you will face.

821. Before you give a directive, decide first if you are prepared to follow through and make your child comply. If you are not going to follow through, then you are better off not giving the directive. Your child will cooperate better if he always sees that you mean what you say.

822. Do not give a directive as a question. If you ask a question, such as "How about cleaning your room now?" you will probably get told just how little she wants to clean her room. If you want your child to clean her room, use a directive: "It is time to clean your room now."

823. It is fine, and even helpful, to add politeness to your directives: "Please use your napkin to wipe your mouth." You're still telling what you want done, not asking.

824. Politeness is not the same as pleading with your child. It is fine to say, "Please," but do not beg for compliance.

825. Do not fall into the trap of giving a directive over and over and over. Give a directive once and wait about ten seconds for compliance. Give it a second time and wait again. The third time, give a warning of the consequence for noncompliance. Instead of asking a fourth time, implement the consequence.

826. Make a list of misbehaviors your child frequently engages in, and write alternative behaviors she should be doing in their place. Try to ignore the misbehaviors and heavily praise the alternative behaviors.

827. Use "When you…, then you…" This will help your child cope with not getting what he wants immediately. If your child asks to watch television, instead of saying "No, it is homework time," say, "When you finish your homework, then you can watch television." Children with ADHD respond better when they know what positive event awaits them after they comply with your directive.

828. Use "I am not saying you can't…" to help avoid a meltdown when you are denying your child's request. Instead of saying, "No, you cannot have a sleepover until you bring up your grades," say, "I am not saying you cannot have a sleepover. What do you think needs to be done before you can have one?"

829. If a behavior is annoying or inappropriate, do not comment on that behavior. Instead, give a directive for an incompatible behavior, one that requires the annoying behavior to stop. "Stop banging your spoon on the table" can be replaced with "Please pass me the salad bowl." Your child has to put the spoon down to pick up the bowl.

830. Teach alternative behaviors of what you want your child to do instead of what she is doing at the moment. Do not do A, do B instead. "Do not throw your clothes on the floor. Put them in your basket instead."

831. Use "If…then…" statements to help your child learn to anticipate the consequences of his behavior. "If you leave your baseball glove on the floor, then the dog will chew it and you won't have a mitt to play with."

832. Instead of saying no, which can result in quick anger outbursts, respond to requests with, "Yes, when…" Finish with what has to happen for the request to be granted. For example: "Yes, you may watch television when you have cleaned your room" or "Yes, you may get a car when you have saved half the money."

833. Increase your child's understanding of why she has to comply with certain directives. If your child resists your direction, nicely ask, "Why do you think I am telling you to do this?" Give her a moment to think about the reason for the behavior. If she cannot come up with a reason, then you can explain it. Children with ADHD will cooperate more if they understand why the particular behavior must be done.

834. Decide which rules are nonnegotiable. Wearing a seat belt, brushing teeth, and leaving the house without permission are examples of rules that have absolutely no room to be negotiated or refused.

835. Hold your child accountable for his behavior. Do not let him use his ADHD as an excuse.

836. Create secret hand signals to use with your child for reminders about what to do. A C shape made with your fingers can remind her to try to remain calm. A finger pointing to your eye can remind her to look. A finger to the ear can be a reminder to listen.

837. Be specific in what you expect from your child's behavior. Telling your child "be good" is vague, and he will not know what you mean by "good." Telling your child, "Stay right next to me in line, and do not leave my side" tells your child exactly what to do.

838. Say it and mean it. Nagging is the fastest way to teach your child you do not mean business and she does not have to do what you say. She will simply have to listen to your annoying lectures, but she still won't have to do what you say.

839. Think of yelling like a delay button. When you become a habitual yeller to get your child to comply, you have taught him that he does not have to do what you say until you reach the point of raising your voice.

840. Build in free playtime each day so your child can play, be loud, run around, and have few rules to follow. When it is time for rules again, it will be easier for your child to cooperate.

841. If your child is not cooperating with certain behaviors or tasks, ask her what would make her motivated to do what you expect of her. You may be pleasantly surprised to learn what small reward she wants in exchange for cooperation.

Tips for
PUNISHMENT

Punishment, if used appropriately, is a highly effective parenting tool for children without ADHD. It seems logical that it should be for children with ADHD too. However, it is just the opposite. Punishment often makes things worse. Children with ADHD, for some reason, do not seem to learn to modify their behavior if they are punished. At best, the punishment has little or no effect. At worst, it causes rage and aggression. Used sparingly, it can be of some help; however, the positive approach has been shown to consistently work better. These eighteen tips will help you use punishment effectively.

842. You can't give a punishment for every misbehavior. ADHD children engage in so many inappropriate behaviors that if you tried to give a punishment for each one, you would be punishing your child all day and night.

843. Use punishment sparingly. Punish only a few misbehaviors that you decide are the most important, and in the meantime, ignore the less important misdeeds or use alternative methods of modifying misbehavior.

844. Earning rewards for cooperating is far more effective in managing behavior problems than punishment.

845. Guide your punishments with the knowledge that ADHD children are far more motivated to earn something than they are to avoid losing something.

846. Each day is a brand new day. Punishments from yesterday are over and your child starts each morning fresh.

847. Spanking a child with ADHD does not make him stop his misbehavior.

848. Punishments longer than one day lose effectiveness because ADHD children quickly lose motivation to behave. If she knows she won't get to play video games for one week, what is going to motivate her to behave?

849. For repeated behaviors that are showing no signs of improvement, double the punishment to make a more dramatic point. Do not go further than double, however, or your child then has lost all incentive to cooperate.

850. Look for a decrease in misbehavior when you use punishment rather than complete disappearance of behavior problems; you won't get it with an ADHD child.

851. Define success in small steps. If your child has five tantrums a day, the goal is for him to have four a day, hold that success for a while, then set a new goal for three a day, hold that success for a while, and so on. You will not go from five tantrums in a day to zero.

852. Make your child earn all privileges. This will motivate your child to cooperate far more than just giving privileges and removing them as a punishment. Television, computer time, and using the phone, for example, are privileges that should be earned.

853. Use logical consequences. Not every misbehavior requires a punishment. If your child refuses to take a coat to school, the logical consequence is that she will be cold. Create logical consequences by thinking about what would happen naturally if you did nothing. Nature will take care of many consequences for you. If your child refuses to eat the lunch you packed, he will go hungry.

854. Everyone wants to be heard and understood. Always

give your child a chance to tell her side of the story before deciding if a punishment is necessary.

855. Mistakes are good teachers. Often a chat with your child about what she can learn from the misdeed is enough to turn the behavior into a permanent lesson without the need for a punishment.

856. What could you do next time? Asking this can help your child use better judgment in the future if he thinks about his behavior. This can be more effective than a punishment.

857. Avoid adding escalating punishments in the midst of a conflict. Adding punishment on top of punishment will result in a desperate child who will get even more out of control.

858. Do not punish crying. Children with ADHD have difficulty soothing themselves and controlling their upset. Threatening to add more punishment if they do not stop crying will result in more crying.

859. If your child also has ODD, punishment will be even less effective. Children with ODD often react to punishment with anger and a desire for revenge against the punishing parent.

Tips for REWARDS

Rewards are your saving grace in raising a child with ADHD. Without rewards, you will struggle with getting your child to do much of anything. Fortunately, most children with ADHD are highly driven to earn rewards. Their personality trait of always wanting more will work to your advantage. These forty-three tips will make managing your child's behavior and getting her to complete her tasks much easier from the moment you put them to use.

860. Understand that children with ADHD need a very high level of motivation to do anything they do not want to do.

861. Start a token economy for your child. Give points or poker chips for every appropriate behavior and task completed, which your child can trade in daily for rewards and privileges.

862. Accept the token economy as your new best friend. Without a structured point system, you have little motivation for your child to comply.

863. Know that giving rewards is not the same as bribing. Rewards are for work well done. Bribes are given when someone does something immoral or illegal in exchange for a reward.

864. Drop the idea that if you give your child rewards, he will never learn to do anything without a reward. Just worry about improving his behavior now.

865. Understand that children with ADHD are not driven by internal rewards of pride and self-satisfaction. Most every child with ADHD will require rewards in exchange for her cooperation and completion of tasks.

866. If you want your child to have the philosophy that those who work hard earn great rewards in life, you have to raise him with rewards for his work now.

867. Do not worry that a token economy will spoil your child. Our entire economy is based on rewards. A paycheck is a reward for showing up to work and doing what you were hired to do. A token economy teaches your child that she will be rewarded for her work, which is to do her best in school and have appropriate behavior.

868. Write out your token economy on a behavior chart that describes what your child is expected to do each day and how many points each behavior and task is worth.

869. Use one chart per week to easily see how the week went.

870. Post the behavior chart where your child can easily see it.

871. Keep a notebook with your behavior charts so you can follow the progress over the months and years.

872. The more severe your child's symptoms, the more behaviors she will have on her list, creating more opportunities for her to earn points.

873. Create a menu of rewards and privileges with your child and assign each a point value. List whatever item and privilege he wants, from a tiny piece of gum or having a sleepover to getting a new bike or taking a trip to Disneyland.

874. Rewards are only motivating if your child is willing to work for them. Make sure the list is made of items and privileges of your child's choice, not yours. You may think that spending a day at the mall is a great idea, but if your child dislikes shopping, it is not a reward.

875. The reward menu should include many items and privileges that can be earned every day, many that take a short while to save for, and some that take a long while to save for.

876. Post the reward menu where your child can easily see it and look to it to motivate her to earn the items and privileges on her list.

877. Continually add to your menu to keep your child motivated to earn new rewards and privileges. The goal is to have enough points earned and enough low-cost rewards and privileges that your child is able to spend points every day. If it is too hard to earn and save points, she will very quickly lose interest.

878. Be aware that children with ADHD have a very hard time delaying gratification and will not be able to wait until the end of the week or month for their reward. Allow your child to spend points every day. You want him to get the idea that if he does well each day, he will be rewarded each day.

879. Be sure to give the rewards and provide the privileges every day regardless of how tired you are. One day of depriving your child of her earned reward or privilege can be enough to destroy the plan.

880. Exceptions to spending points include serious problems, such as being suspended from school. Your child can still earn points on his suspension days but may not spend any.

881. Assign a monetary value to each point so your child can save up points to buy items or activities she wants. One to five cents per point is reasonable. Consider your budget for rewards and assign points accordingly. If she wants a $20 item, consider how often you can afford it, but do not make it more than once per week, even if you can easily afford it.

882. Do not make it too easy or too hard for him to save enough points to buy something. You want your child to work for his rewards, but not to have to wait so long that he loses motivation.

883. If your child wants an expensive item put on her

reward list, add it no matter what it costs. Simply assign the appropriate point value to it. It may take six months or six years for her to save enough points.

884. Regardless of how much money you have to spend on rewards, do not overindulge your child. All children need to know the value of working and saving for things they want.

885. Make the amount of money you spend on rewards age-appropriate. A $100 shopping spree is not appropriate for an elementary school child but might be for a high school teen.

886. Realize that overindulgence in rewards deprives your child of learning how to delay gratification.

887. Rewards do not have to cost money; in fact, most of them should be free or very low-cost. Many things you automatically give your child can be turned into rewards. Watching movies, going out for pizza, eating dessert, trips to the park, staying up late, etc., can all be rewards that cost no more than you are already spending.

888. Everything other than food, adequate clothing, shelter, and health care can be used as a reward. Special play time with parents, taking a walk with Mom, riding a bike with Dad, or playing board games with both parents are all examples of free rewards your child can earn.

889. Making fun activities involving time with a parent a reward, rather than an automatic right, will help you and your child spend more time together. Most children with ADHD are hungry for special time alone with their parents and are motivated to work hard to earn it.

890. Points can be spent only after homework is done.

891. Screen time with computers, video games, and television is a reward, not an inalienable right, and should be earned. A general rule of thumb is ten points per half hour.

892. Using a point system teaches your child how to set priorities on his free time. If he were allowed to watch unlimited TV, he probably would spend hours on end doing so. If he must choose how to spend his points, he is far more likely to choose to watch less TV and spend his points on other rewards and privileges or engage in activities that are always free, such as reading.

893. Set a limit on how much screen time your child is

allowed on school days and weekends. Just because she has one hundred points saved does not mean she can spend it all on five hours of nonstop video games.

894.   Rewards teach your child to be careful about material goods. He may want every toy he sees and demand each one if he is accustomed to getting everything he wants. If he is taught to save his points and use them on items he wants and can afford, he will be more selective, less demanding, and more appreciative of the items he earns.

895.   Be somewhat liberal in allowing your child to spend his points on privileges. While no parent really wants his child to watch a lot of television or eat a lot of candy, these can be exceedingly powerful motivators that can dramatically increase your child's cooperation.

896.   Give plenty of bonus points. Any extra task done without being asked, any kindness shown, any chores done without a reminder are all worthy of bonus points. A good standard is five bonus points per task or kindness shown.

897.   Give an abundance of points. You want your child to learn from the point program "do good, get good." Be generous, and create easy ways for your child to earn points.

898. Tasks that are done without any prompt earn four bonus points, plus one point for doing the task.

899. Tasks that are done with only one prompt earn three bonus points, plus one point for doing the task.

900. Tasks that require more than one prompt earn only one point.

901. Tasks not done earn zero points.

902. Do not remove points already earned. While this strategy can work for nondisordered children, it can be a disaster for ADHD children. Removing points already earned results in anger, frustration, and a loss of motivation to keep trying hard to earn more.

903. Do not create inflation by raising the cost of rewards and privileges. This will make your child lose motivation and ruin your token economy.

Tips for TANTRUMS

Tantrums can occur in ADHD children long after the toddler years are over. While tantrums appear to be a strong-willed child's way of getting what he wants, recent studies suggest that children with ADHD lack the brain development that allows them to calm themselves down. If parents work from this hypothesis rather than assuming that the child is manipulating, then more effective strategies can be used. Use these twenty-eight tips to manage and decrease tantrums.

904. Do not regard tantrums as purposeful plots to manipulate you. Children with ADHD often have tantrums because they lack the brain development to manage their upset emotions.

905. Ignore tantrums as often as you can. Ignore means not looking at, touching, or talking to your child while she is having a tantrum.

906. While ignoring a tantrum, be sure that there is no danger to your child. If you need to protect his safety, do so, but then return to ignoring until he stops.

907. Do not try to reason with your child during a tantrum. In the midst of a tantrum, the emotional part of your child's brain is directing her behavior and she is not able to use the logical part.

908. Avoid a lecture or long talk after a tantrum. Get back to business as usual as soon as your child calms down. You want him to learn that once he calms down, everything goes back to normal, and the sooner he calms down, the sooner things get back on track.

909. Return to the situation or directive that caused the tantrum as soon as it is over. If your child has a tantrum because you said it was time to take a bath, once her tantrum is over, repeat the directive, "Now it is time for your bath." You want her to learn that a tantrum does not mean that she gets out of doing what is expected of her.

910. Do not physically try to stop a tantrum. If your child tears apart her room during a tantrum, let it happen, unless there is a danger to him or you. Ignore it, and when his tantrum is over and he has cooperated with the initial directive that caused the tantrum, then he must clean his room.

911.   Do not replace unnecessary items destroyed in a tantrum. Your child needs to learn that if she breaks her items, she loses them.

912.   Have your child replace any necessary items broken in a tantrum. He can pay with his money or work off the cost with chores.

913.   Be prepared that when you begin to ignore tantrums, they will become more intense and last longer. This is your child's way of trying to get you to react and give in. Ride it out, and as long as she is safe, let the tantrum play itself out so she learns that she won't get her way by having a meltdown.

914.   Leave the room during a tantrum, providing safety is not an issue. A tantrum is useless unless someone is there to watch it. If you leave the room, your child loses his audience. He may follow you around, but you can continue about your business.

915.   Offer an alternative behavior your child can engage in once she quits the tantrum. "When you are done with your tantrum, you can return to the table and finish your dinner."

916. Keep a log of how long tantrums last and how often they occur so you can monitor if your responses are helping. Do not let your child know you are doing this; it is for your knowledge, not your child's.

917. Direct your child to stop his tantrum or else he can go to his room until he is finished.

918. Get back to normal after a tantrum. You do not want your child to learn that tantrums are followed by excessive positive attention. Do not withhold normal attention, but do not engage in a special cuddle session afterward.

919. Do not make any threats of punishment during a tantrum. This only adds to your child's upset and anger and escalates the meltdown.

920. Do not assume your child is purposely having a tantrum to manipulate you. This will only make you angry and decrease your ability to stay calm and use your ignoring skills.

921. Try to prevent tantrums by talking about the problem.

When your child looks on the verge of a tantrum, prompt him by saying, "Tell me what's making you upset and let's see what we can do about it."

922. Prevent future tantrums by praising your child when she properly handles her upset. "I like the way you told me you were mad about not getting to stay up late. You handled that really well!"

923. Be certain that you are not having adult tantrums when you are upset. Your child will learn how to express and keep his feelings under proper control by watching and listening to how you handle your upset.

924. Do not do your child's chores if she has a tantrum. If she has a tantrum because she does not want to clean up her toys, resist the temptation to clean them up yourself; otherwise, she learns a tantrum means you do the chores.

925. Do not give in to a tantrum. If you said no, stick with it, no matter how intense the tantrum is or how much you feel your child has worn you down. If you give in, you only have yourself to blame for the next tantrum; after all, you are the one who taught your child that if he has a tantrum long enough, he will eventually get his way.

926. You can't stop a tantrum. Only your child can stop it.

927. Know that there is nothing you can do to *make* your child stop screaming or crying, so do not try.

928. Avoid tantrums by not placing your child in situations that are high-risk for a meltdown. If you know your child has a tantrum almost every time you take her to the grocery store, alter your schedule and find a time when your child does not have to accompany you.

929. Prevent tantrums by bringing your "tantrum prevention kit." Put in the kit items you know are likely to keep your child happy and calm, such as snacks, drinks, toys, books, music, etc.

930. Know your child's limits and plan accordingly. Keep a log of situations that result in tantrums so you can learn what sets your child off. Avoid or alter the situation so you can prevent upset.

931. Control your emotions during a tantrum. Your child will not be able to control her emotions if yours are out of control.

Tips for
TIME MANAGEMENT

Children with ADHD have a very poor concept of time. Tasks that are boring seem to last an eternity to them, causing dawdling, procrastination, and a variety of ways to attempt to escape. Some children will spend more time procrastinating than it would take to just get the task done. Fun activities always end too fast, causing emotional meltdowns when it is time to stop. Managing time is a frontal lobe task that the majority of children with ADHD do not do well. Parents must be their surrogate frontal lobe and keep track of time for their child for many years past what they might expect. Fortunately, you have these twelve tips to give you some assistance.

932. Understand that children with ADHD have a poor concept of time. Even after they are well able to read a clock, they are poor at estimating time and very poor at monitoring how much time is passing as they engage in a task.

933. Use a watch with multiple timers to prompt your child to engage in scheduled tasks.

934. Post a weekly schedule on your child's wall that lists her tasks to be done and when they need to be completed.

935. Do not expect a task to be completed unless it is listed on the schedule. Be sure to include ordinary tasks of waking up, eating, brushing teeth, getting in the car for school, homework time, free time, bath time, etc.

936. Start to teach your child how to monitor time by playing a "beat the clock game" for short tasks. Set a timer and challenge your child to make her bed, for example, before the timer goes off. She can earn points for making her bed and bonus points if she beats the clock.

937. Help your child learn to estimate time by playing a game of "guess how long it will take." Challenge your child to guess how long it will take him to put away all his toys in his toy box. Set the stopwatch and time him. He can earn points for completing the task and bonus points if he does it faster or within one minute of his guess.

938. Let your child time you while you do tasks. She will learn time management from watching you try to "beat the clock."

939. Post a schedule on the wall with a picture of each task to be completed alongside a picture of a clock showing what time it needs to be done by.

940. Make a task board with two columns, one for "to do" and one for "done." Make task cards for your child to move from the "to do" column to the "done" column when he has completed each one. Task boards can be made with felt, using Velcro to attach the task cards, a dry-erase board using magnet strips on which you can write the task, or a paper chart with magnets posted on the refrigerator.

941. Monitor how long each task takes your child to complete and modify as needed. If tasks are taking longer than you originally thought they would, change the schedule so your child can achieve success.

942. Your child may need you to stand nearby while she does her tasks. This is true of young children and of most children with ADHD. If your child repeatedly is unable to complete a project on her own, this is your cue that she needs your presence and directions to help get tasks done in a timely manner.

943. Give countdown reminders so your child knows how much time is left to complete a given task. Ten-, five-, and one-minute countdowns are helpful.

Tips for MARRIAGE

Pay attention to how your child's ADHD is impacting your marriage. By the time an ADHD child is eight years old, his parents are twice as likely to divorce as those of an eight-year-old child without ADHD. These eighteen tips can help you so you do not become a statistic.

944. Your child's other parent is your partner in the success and happiness of your child.

945. The only way to raise a child with ADHD is by team parenting.

946. If your spouse has trouble with your child, even if you think nothing is wrong with your child, you still must join your spouse's parenting team and work together.

947. Put effort into keeping your marriage positive. Vow not to let parenting struggles negatively impact your marriage.

948. Both parents should be involved in their child's life, even if one of you does not agree with the diagnosis of ADHD.

949. Remind yourself that your spouse did not cause your child to have ADHD—even if your spouse has it too.

950. Fighting about your child's behavior is a clear sign that you do not have an agreed upon method for handling misbehavior.

951. Plan some weekly time away from your child, even if it is talking together in the backyard while the children are watching television.

952. Take turns having free adult time so each parent gets to have some time away from children, home, and responsibilities, even for just a few hours.

953. Take turns with child duties so neither parent gets burned out taking care of the same task over and over.

954. Act like a team, even if you are not in agreement with a particular decision the other parent makes. When you have private time, you can talk about how you would have handled it.

955. You were a couple before you were parents; remember to be a couple after you have children.

956. Get someone to watch the children and go on a date.

957. Learn about ADHD together. The more knowledge you both have, the easier the parenting will be.

958. Do not leave the parenting to the other parent. Do your share.

959. Promise that your child's behavior will not be a source of conflict in your marriage, but instead just a problem for which together you need to find a solution.

960. View your spouse as a partner in the business of raising your child.

961. Divorced parents are still partners in raising their child and should participate equally.

Tips for VACATIONS

Time off from school can be the happiest time in the lives of families living with ADHD. The stress of having to get up early, be in school, do homework, and get to bed on time all disappear when school's out. However, even though your child is on vacation, his symptoms are not. These thirty-three tips will give you plenty of ways to make vacations the happiest time of the year.

962. Talk to your child's teacher about not assigning work over vacation periods. Adults do not have to work during their vacations; why should children? Vacations are a time of planned relaxation, fun, and time away from the ordinary stresses and tasks of daily life and therefore should be free of work, including homework and school projects.

963. When planning vacation time, consider how your child functions best. Is he better behaved when he has numerous structured activities to keep him occupied, or does he seem more relaxed and calm when he has plenty of free time to just play without too many limits imposed on him?

964. If taking a road trip, schedule longer rest stops than you would if you were alone. Instead of eating at a restaurant where your child has to sit and contain himself, consider getting food to go and finding a park to have a picnic so you can let your child run around for a while.

965. If you prefer your child has some time away from technology on your road trip, plan some fun old-fashioned road games like alphabet or license plate games.

966. Keep your child occupied and free from boredom with a book on CD that she can listen to with headphones or the family can enjoy through the car stereo.

967. When traveling on an airplane, pack multiple items for entertainment. Take into account that a three-hour flight involves about seven hours of time, including getting to the airport, parking, check-in, security, waiting, boarding, waiting for takeoff, flight time, disembarking, walking to and waiting for luggage, and transportation to your destination. This is a long time for your child to keep himself in control under the stressful circumstances of air travel.

968. Bring quiet activities for airplane flights that do not disturb other passengers, such as video games with the mute button on, a DVD player with headphones, word search puzzles, comic books, etc.

969. When selecting which type of vacation you will take, consider how your child will behave. An excessively hyperactive child will probably not do well on a group tour where you have to consider other travelers. A loud, easily bored child will probably not do well with a museum tour.

970. Be aware that your child will enjoy a vacation more, and therefore have better behavior, if the vacation involves a favorite topic or activity. Children interested in space would enjoy visiting Kennedy Space Center in Florida or the National Air and Space Museum in Washington, D.C.; those interested in sea mammals would enjoy a trip to SeaWorld.

971. Be sure to schedule "free time" on your vacation so your child has opportunities to play, relax, read, etc.

972. Ask your child to contribute to the list of family rules for vacation. Be ready to suggest categories such as airport behavior, airplane behavior, car behavior, waiting in line behavior, Grandma's house behavior, etc. If the rules are "family rules" instead of rules just for the children, you will likely gain more cooperation, since your child will be more willing to follow the rules if you have to follow them too.

973. Consider how much screen time you will allow your child to have during vacation. You can be generous and allow more time than during school periods, but unlimited use of video games, computers, and television is not a good idea even on vacation.

974. Choose family-friendly hotels so you won't be worried about upsetting or distracting other guests, which in turn upsets you and your child.

975. Choose a hotel with a pool so your child can burn up energy and have fun at the same time.

976. For very active children, consider a vigorous physical activity to burn off some energy before your main activity of the day. An hour swim in the pool will make the trip to the museum less hectic.

977. Pack your children's suitcases with complete outfits packed in individual large plastic bags. Include socks, a shirt, pants, underwear, a jacket, etc. Your child will be able to dress quickly, and his suitcase will stay organized.

978. Your teen will want to pack for herself. Let her lay out everything she plans to take and go over it with her so she has another set of eyes to see if she is bringing enough or too much. Check her choices for their appropriateness for the weather, activity, and cultural environment.

979. Choose child-centered vacations so you and your children have fun. Cruise ships, hotels, and resorts that cater to families are good choices.

980. Choose daily activities that are child-centered. A day of wine tasting in the vineyards is sure to be a disaster, while a day at the beach guarantees fun for almost any child.

981. Decrease boredom by choosing activities where your child has something to do. A nature hike might be boring and tiring for some children, but if your child participates in the Junior Ranger program, she will likely be more interested and enjoy herself. Museum exhibits might be dull unless your son can get his museum passport book stamped.

982. Create your own game for your child to do when

visiting attractions that might not hold her interest. Visiting an art museum might be terribly boring, but if your child is assigned to count how many babies are in all the paintings you see, she might be more eager to enjoy herself instead of complain.

983. Make your own trivia game when visiting attractions. Look on the Internet or in a guidebook for facts that you will learn at the attraction. Type several questions on a colorful piece of paper, and when you arrive at the destination, you can give your child the trivia game. Promise a treat at the end of the visit if he gets all the questions correct (be sure to help him!). A visit to Kennedy Space Center might have questions such as "What was the name of the first chimp in space?" "Who was the first man to walk on the moon?" and "What is the longest time man has spent in space?"

984. Do not plan too many activities in one day.

985. If there is any chance of getting separated from your child, take walkie-talkies for instant communication.

986. Define boundaries of where your child can go and where she cannot cross.

987. Arm your child with an ID that has his name, your name, and your cell phone number. ROAD ID offers custom engraved bracelets for $16.

988. Expect some meltdowns and try not to view them as ruining your trip. Travel can make everyone cranky. Be patient, let the meltdown melt, and when it is over, carry on.

989. Carry poker chips with you to give to your child anytime she does something "chip worthy," such as something kind, helpful, or appropriate without being asked. On the last day of the trip, she can trade the chips in for money to buy a souvenir. Depending on how long the trip is and how many points you expect her to earn, set the cash value of the chips ahead of time at one, five, ten, or twenty-five cents per chip.

990. Instead of poker chips, give your child a small spiral notepad and pen where he can keep track of his "chip-worthy" points. He will enjoy putting the marks in each time he earns a chip or a point. As the trip goes on, he will be pleased with himself each time he tallies up his growing number of points.

991. If you child's vacation time will be spent at home, plan special activities for you and your child to engage in to make the time off stand out as a fun and special time of the year. This will make your child's vacation more enjoyable and can motivate her to do her best during the school year, knowing that she has many special activities to look forward to.

992. For vacation time at home, consider if your child will do better at home with freedom and limited structure, or does he require a highly structured day camp where he is kept occupied and supervised all day?

993. Create a stay-at-home vacation schedule, but be flexible about it. Your child will function better if there is some structure set into her day. She can sleep later than usual and eat breakfast in her PJs, but she should still get up by a certain time each day, eat before going out to play, have lunch and dinner at a relatively set time period, and have a later but still set bedtime.

994. If your child will be attending a camp on vacation, consider the camp's ability to effectively work with your child. If your child has behavioral challenges, be sure to interview the camp director about the staff's experience, ability, and willingness to work with children with ADHD.

Tips for OTHER PEOPLE'S OPINIONS

ADHD is a hot topic these days, and it seems that everyone has an opinion about it. Many people have opinions about you, your child, and how you should parent. It is easy to become upset and feel like you have to defend yourself. Knowing that you will surely be faced with unwanted advice, here are nine tips to help you take control of the conversation.

995. Decide who you should tell about your child's ADHD. If your child only has difficulty with school and homework issues, but is free of noticeable behavior problems, then there is no point in risking embarrassing her and telling others about her school issues.

996. Consider telling others if your child is hyperactive, loud, impulsive, and has trouble cooperating. Other adults will notice your child's behavior rather quickly anyway, so it can help to disclose your child's ADHD up front. You are less likely to be judged harshly and more likely to receive support if you disclose.

997. Disclose that your child has ADHD to any adult whose home your child will be visiting. It is fair to the other family and to your child. Tell the adults the necessary information they need to know about your child to help the visit go well.

998. Telling your relatives and friends about your child's ADHD can save you from having to hear their criticism, advice, or comments, such as "If he were my child, he would never act that way!"

999. Anticipate that relatives and friends may give their opinions, advice, wisdom, and even criticism about your child's behavior and the way you handle it. Prepare ahead of time a gracious way of responding that will not cause a conflict but, at the same time, politely lets the other person know you have it under control. For example: "Thanks for that idea; I will give it some serious thought."

1000. If you have people in your life who always seem to give unsolicited advice, consider beating them to the punch by letting them know you see the problems, you are working on them, and the situation is not open to discussion. For example, "We are very much looking forward to seeing you. As you know, Nicholas has ADHD and can be rather hyperactive, especially when he is in new places. He might behave in ways that are different from other kids you know. We are working with a psychologist who has us using specific methods, so I want to assure you that I will take care of any behavioral issues Nicholas might have while we are at your house."

1001. Anticipate that people will argue with you about your child's diagnosis being an excuse or a made-up disorder, that if you just were a better disciplinarian, he would not act this way. Prepare a graceful response that won't start a debate, but instead will tactfully communicate that this topic is not open for discussion. For example: "I know how you feel, Uncle Bobby. Many people think the same thing. Regardless of whether you think ADHD is real, we can all see that Matthew has some challenges, and we are working on them."

1002. Expect to hear opinions about medication, both vehemently for and against. You do not have to disclose whether you are medicating or defend your decision. You can cut short the conversation with a closing remark, such as "Thanks for sharing your thoughts; I know many people share your viewpoint" or "I like your passion about your opinion."

1003. Do consider listening to the opinions and advice of others. Even if someone is judging you or has opinions that are contrary to yours, she still might have something valuable to say.

Resources

Bedtime
- toolsforwellness.com: Harmonic Sleep CD
- hemi-sync.com: Hemi-sync's Sound Sleeper CD
- Sleepsonic.com: Pillowsonic Pillow

Fidgeting
- Tanglecreations.com: small, colorful, quiet fidget toys
- Wikkistix.com: small, quiet fidget toys

Focus
- Simplynoise.com: white noise machines
- whitenoiseforfree.com: white noise headsets

Getting Ready for School
- Sunrise System Dawn Simulator: gradual light alarm clock
- Underarmour.com: soft undergarments to prevent irritation from clothing
- softclothing.net: Clothing for children with tactile sensitivities
- Smartknitkids.com: seamless socks

- Tictactoe.net: seamless socks
- Towelspa Towel Warmer: small, portable towel warmer

Homework

- Headsupnow.com: supplies information for parents and teachers for children with ADHD
- Abledata.com: talking calculator that speaks the number and symbol pushed
- www.eudesign.com/mnems: common mnenonics to help with memorization

Math

- *Times Tables the Fun Way*: books filled with fun memory and visual tricks to help children learn multiplication tables
- Citycreek.com: fun ways to learn math
- TeaChildMath.com: workbook that uses fun visual tricks and patterns to help your child memorize his multiplication tables

Organization

- EZ-Find! Item Wireless Locator: provides 25 colored fobs and a remote
- Stickies: a computer program that looks just like Post-its that sit on the desktop so they can't be missed

Reading

- Learningally.org: Learning Ally, formerly Recording for the Blind & Dyslexic, offers almost any book on tape/CD. These are available free to anyone with vision or reading problems.
- National Library Service (www.loc.gov/nls): offers almost any book on tape/CD free

Special Education

- Wrightslaw.com: information about special education
- *The ADD & ADHD Answer Book: Professional Answers to the Top 275 Questions Parents Ask* by Susan Ashley, PhD, Sourcebooks 2005
- COPPA.org (Council of Parent Attorneys and Advocates): resources to find special education attorneys and advocates

Time Management

- Watchminder.com: WatchMinder allows you to set thirty alarms per day with beeps and/or vibration along with written messages reminding your child what to do, such as take medications, use the restroom, pay attention, etc.
- Timelymatters.com: On Task On Time is as much a toy as a timer, and thus younger children will be eager to use it. Select the activity, put the proper sticker with a picture of the task, and set the timer.

- Timetimer.com: The Time Timer covers the face of the clock and shows only how much time is left, thereby removing the distraction of the entire clock.

Vacations

- RoadID.com: IDs you can customize and wear on your arm, neck, or shoe

About the Author

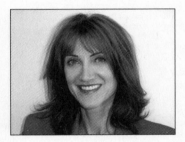

Susan Ashley, PhD, author of *The ADD & ADHD Answer Book* and *The Asperger's Syndrome Answer Book*, is the founder and director of Ashley Children's Psychology Center in Los Angeles, CA. She has specialized in ADHD since 1990. A graduate of UCLA and California School of Professional Psychology, she has more than twenty-five years of education, training, and experience working with children and families. She has lectured extensively across the United States on childhood psychological disorders, including ADHD, ODD, OCD, Tourette's, and Asperger's. Dr. Ashley also practices forensic psychology and serves as an expert witness in juvenile and adult cases in civil, family, and criminal court.

Have a tip that works? Send your tips to bestadhdtips@ me.com. Dr. Ashley will post tips anonymously on her website at www.ashleypsychology.com.